Michael T. Wright
B. R. Simon Rosser
Onno de Zwart
Editors

New International Directions in HIV Prevention for Gay and Bisexual Men

New International Directions in HIV Prevention for Gay and Bisexual Men has been co-published simultaneously as *Journal of Psychology & Human Sexuality*, Volume 10, Numbers 3/4 1998.

Pre-publication REVIEWS, COMMENTARIES, EVALUATIONS . . .

"**P**erforms a great service to HIV prevention research and health promotion. . . . It takes the words of gay and bisexual men seriously by locating men's sexual practice in their love relationships and casual sex encounters and examines their response to HIV."

Susan Kippax
*Associate Professor and Director
National Centre in HIV Social Research
School of Behavioural Sciences
Macquarie University
New South Wales, Australia*

New International Directions in HIV Prevention for Gay and Bisexual Men

New International Directions in HIV Prevention for Gay and Bisexual Men has been co-published simultaneously as *Journal of Psychology & Human Sexuality*, Volume 10, Numbers 3/4 1998.

New International Directions in HIV Prevention for Gay and Bisexual Men

Michael T. Wright, LICSW
B. R. Simon Rosser, PhD, MPH
Onno de Zwart, MA
Editors

New International Directions in HIV Prevention for Gay and Bisexual Men edited by Michael T. Wright, B. R. Simon Rosser, and Onno de Zwart, was simultaneously issued by The Haworth Press, Inc., under the same title, as a special issue of *Journal of Psychology & Human Sexuality*, Volume 10, Numbers 3/4, Eli Coleman, Editor.

Harrington Park Press
An Imprint of
The Haworth Press, Inc.
New York • London

ISBN 1-56023-116-5

Published by

Harrrington Park Press, 10 Alice Street, Binghamton, NY 13904-1580 USA

Harrrington Park Press is an imprint of The Haworth Press, Inc., 10 Alice Street, Binghamton, NY 13904-1580 USA.

New International Directions in HIV Prevention for Gay and Bisexual Men has been co-published simultaneously as *Journal of Psychology & Human Sexuality*™, Volume 10, Numbers 3/4 1998.

© 1998 by The Haworth Press, Inc. All rights reserved. No part of this work may be reproduced or utilized in any form or by any means, electronic or mechanical, including photocopying, microfilm and recording, or by any information storage and retrieval system, without permission in writing from the publisher. Printed in the United States of America.

The development, preparation, and publication of this work has been undertaken with great care. However, the publisher, employees, editors, and agents of The Haworth Press and all imprints of The Haworth Press, Inc., including The Haworth Medical Press® and Pharmaceutical Products Press®, are not responsible for any errors contained herein or for consequences that may ensue from use of materials or information contained in this work. Opinions expressed by the author(s) are not necessarily those of The Haworth Press, Inc.

Cover design by Monica Seifert

Library of Congress Cataloging-in-Publication Data

New international directions in HIV prevention for gay and bisexual men / Michael T. Wright, B. R. Simon Rosser, Onno de Zwart, editors.
    p. cm.
    "New international directions in HIV prevention for gay and bisexual men has been co-published simultaneously as Journal of psychology & human sexuality, Volume 10, Numbers 3/4 1998."
    Includes bibliographical references and index.
    ISBN 0-7890-0538-7 (alk. paper).–ISBN 1-56023-116-5 (alk. paper).
    1. Gay men–Sexual behavior. 2. Bisexual men–Sexual behavior. 3. AIDS (Disease)–Prevention. I. Wright, Michael T. II. Rosser, B. R. Simon. III. Zwart, Onno de. IV. Journal of psychology & human sexuality.
HQ76.N48 1998
306.76'6–dc21
                                                      98-27620
                                                          CIP

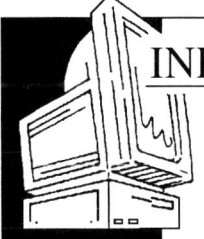

INDEXING & ABSTRACTING

Contributions to this publication are selectively indexed or abstracted in print, electronic, online, or CD-ROM version(s) of the reference tools and information services listed below. This list is current as of the copyright date of this publication. See the end of this section for additional notes.

- *Biology Digest,* Plexus Publishing Company, 143 Old Marlton Pike, Medford, NJ 08055-8750

- *Cambridge Scientific Abstracts,* 7200 Wisconsin Avenue #601, Bethesda, MD 20814

- *CNPIEC Reference Guide: Chinese National Directory of Foreign Periodicals,* P.O. Box 88, Beijing, People's Republic of China

- *Digest of Neurology and Psychiatry,* The Institute of Living, 400 Washington Street, Hartford, CT 06106

- *Educational Administration Abstracts (EAA),* Sage Publications, Inc., 2455 Teller Road, Newbury Park, CA 91320

- *Family Studies Database (online and CD/ROM),* National Information Services Corporation, 306 East Baltimore Pike, 2nd Floor, Media, PA 19063

- *Family Violence & Sexual Assault Bulletin,* Family Violence & Sexual Assault Institute, 1121 E South East Loop #323, Suite 130, Tyler, TX 75701

- *Higher Education Abstracts,* Claremont Graduate University, 231 East Tenth Street, Claremont, CA 91711

- *IBZ International Bibliography of Periodical Literature,* Zeller Verlag GmbH & Co., P.O.B. 1949, D-49009 Osnabruck, Germany

- *Index to Periodical Articles Related to Law,* University of Texas, 727 East 26th Street, Austin, TX 78705

(continued)

- *INTERNET ACCESS (& additional networks) Bulletin Board for Libraries ("BUBL") coverage of information resources on INTERNET, JANET, and other networks.*
    - <URL:http://bubl.ac.uk/>
    - The new locations will be found under <URL:http://bubl.ac.uk/link/>.
    - Any existing BUBL users who have problems finding information on the new service should contact the BUBL help line by sending e-mail to <bubl@bubl.ac.uk>.
  The Andersonian Library, Curran Building, 101 St. James Road, Glasgow G4 0NS, Scotland
- *Mental Health Abstracts (online through DIALOG),* IFI/Plenum Data Company, 3202 Kirkwood Highway, Wilmington, DE 19808
- *Periodica Islamica,* Berita Publishing, 22 Jalan Liku, 59100 Kuala Lumpur, Malaysia
- *Psychological Abstracts (PsycINFO),* American Psychological Association, P.O. Box 91600, Washington, DC 20090-1600
- *Referativnyi Zhurnal (Abstracts Journal of the All-Russian Institute of Scientific and Technical Information),* 20 Usievich Street, Moscow 125219, Russia
- *Sage Family Studies Abstracts (SFSA),* Sage Publications, Inc., 2455 Teller Road, Newbury Park, CA 91320
- *Sage Urban Studies Abstracts (SUSA),* Sage Publications, Inc., 2455 Teller Road, Newbury Park, CA 91320
- *Social Planning/Policy & Development Abstracts (SOPODA),* Sociological Abstracts, Inc., P.O. Box 22206, San Diego, CA 92192-0206
- *Social Work Abstracts,* National Association of Social Workers, 750 First Street NW, 8th Floor, Washington, DC 20002
- *Sociological Abstracts (SA),* Sociological Abstracts, Inc., P.O. Box 22206, San Diego, CA 92192-0206
- *Studies on Women Abstracts,* Carfax Publishing Company, P.O. Box 25, Abingdon, Oxon OX14 3UE, United Kingdom
- *Violence and Abuse Abstracts: A Review of Current Literature on Interpersonal Violence (VAA),* Sage Publications, Inc., 2455 Teller Road, Newbury Park, CA 91320

(continued)

SPECIAL BIBLIOGRAPHIC NOTES

*related to special journal issues (separates)
and indexing/abstracting*

- ❑ indexing/abstracting services in this list will also cover material in any "separate" that is co-published simultaneously with Haworth's special thematic journal issue or DocuSerial. Indexing/abstracting usually covers material at the article/chapter level.

- ❑ monographic co-editions are intended for either non-subscribers or libraries which intend to purchase a second copy for their circulating collections.

- ❑ monographic co-editions are reported to all jobbers/wholesalers/approval plans. The source journal is listed as the "series" to assist the prevention of duplicate purchasing in the same manner utilized for books-in-series.

- ❑ to facilitate user/access services all indexing/abstracting services are encouraged to utilize the co-indexing entry note indicated at the bottom of the first page of each article/chapter/contribution.

- ❑ this is intended to assist a library user of any reference tool (whether print, electronic, online, or CD-ROM) to locate the monographic version if the library has purchased this version but not a subscription to the source journal.

- ❑ individual articles/chapters in any Haworth publication are also available through the Haworth Document Delivery Service (HDDS).

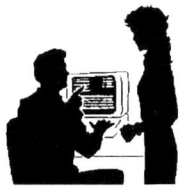

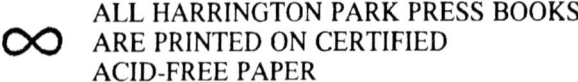

ALL HARRINGTON PARK PRESS BOOKS
ARE PRINTED ON CERTIFIED
ACID-FREE PAPER

CONTENTS

Preface	xiii
Acknowledgments	xvii
The Chorin Document: A Joint Statement of Recommendations for HIV Prevention Targeting Men Who Have Sex with Men *Michael T. Wright, LICSW, MS*	1
Beyond Risk Factors: Trends in European Safer Sex Research *Michael T. Wright, LICSW, MS*	7
Not All Men, Situations, and Actions Are Equal: Moving from 100% Protection to a More Realistic Prevention Practice *Marie-Ange Schiltz, MA*	19
The Importance of Contextualizing Research: An Analysis of Data from the German Gay Press Surveys *Michael Bochow, PhD*	37
Gay Men and HIV: Community Responses and Personal Risks *Peter Keogh, BA* *Susan Beardsell, PhD* *Peter Davies, PhD* *Ford Hickson, BSc* *Peter Weatherburn, MSc*	59
In This Together: The Limits of Prevention Based on Self-Interest and the Role of Altruism in HIV Safety *David Nimmons, BA*	75

Anal Sex and Gay Men: The Challenge of HIV
and Beyond   89
    Onno de Zwart, MA
    Marty P. N. van Kerkhof, MA
    Theo G. M. Sandfort, PhD

Imaginary Protections Against AIDS   103
    Rommel Mendès-Leite, PhD

Desire, Cultural Dissonance, and Incentives
for Remaining HIV-Negative   123
    Wayne Blankenship, MA

Context Is Everything: Thoughts on Effective
HIV Prevention and Gay Men in the United States   133
    Eric Rofes, MA

The Impact of New Advances in Treatment on HIV
Prevention: Implications of the XI International
AIDS Conference on Future Prevention Directions   143
    B. R. Simon Rosser, PhD, MPH

The Impact of New Treatments and Other Trends
on HIV Prevention for Gay and Bisexual Men
in the United States: Observations from the 19th National
Lesbian and Gay Health Association Conference   151
    B. R. Simon Rosser, PhD, MPH
    Michael T. Wright, LICSW, MS

Authors' Notes   159

Index   163

ABOUT THE EDITORS

Michael T. Wright, LICSW, MS, served as a consultant and Director of International Relations at the Deutsche AIDS-Hilfe, the national German AIDS organization, from 1994-1997. Involved with HIV prevention work since 1984, he has served as a consultant, workshop leader, clinical supervisor, and psychotherapist. Wright is a graduate of the Harvard School of Public Health and is currently conducting research at the Institute for Prevention and Psychosocial Research at The Free University in Berlin, Germany.

B. R. Simon Rosser, PhD, MPH, is Associate Professor and licensed psychologist in the Program in Human Sexuality, Department of Family Practice and Community Health, at the Medical School of the University of Minnesota in Minneapolis. He is the author of two books and numerous articles on aspects of HIV prevention and human sexuality. In addition, Dr. Rosser serves on the Minnesota Health Commissioner's Task Force on HIV and STD prevention. Currently, he is principal investigator of a study funded by the Centers for Disease Control that is examining new approaches to HIV prevention targeting gay and bisexual men.

Onno de Zwart, MA, is HIV/AIDS Policy Coordinator at the Rotterdam Municipal Health Service in the Netherlands. As a former researcher in the Department of Gay and Lesbian Studies at Utrecht University, he focused on the sexual behavior of gay and bisexual men and on Dutch HIV prevention policy.

Preface

There is broad consensus within the HIV/AIDS prevention community that new models are needed to address the challenges faced by prevention work at this stage in the epidemic. The current situation in most countries presents us with new challenges to find ways to communicate effectively and to create change within an increasingly diverse array of settings and cultural groups. The question is: Where do we stand in our current theory and practice and where do we need to go in developing the next generation of prevention strategies? In this collection, we ask specifically: What are the next steps in designing effective prevention for gay and bisexual men?

Although there is considerable discussion in the professional journals concerning the various problems confronting HIV/AIDS prevention, there is a need to focus and intensify the debate so as to encourage innovation at both the practical and theoretical levels. To achieve this end, the Deutsche AIDS-Hilfe (DAH), the national German AIDS organization, sponsored a unique series of symposia in 1996 to promote international collaboration in the development of new paradigms for thinking about sexuality and HIV prevention. This resulted in a sort of traveling colloquium being created, with theorists and practitioners from Europe and North America meeting in Germany, Canada, and the United States. Specifically, the three symposia were held in: Chorin, Germany in May 1996 in conjunction with a national German prevention conference; in Seattle in July as part of the American National Lesbian and Gay Health Conference/National AIDS/HIV Forum; and in Vancouver, Canada in July as a satellite meeting at the XI International AIDS Conference. For this volume we have asked some of the symposia participants to share their thoughts so as to make the results of these exciting meetings available to an even larger audience.

[Haworth co-indexing entry note]: "Preface." Wright, Michael T., B. R. Simon Rosser, and Onno de Zwart. Co-published simultaneously in *Journal of Psychology & Human Sexuality* (The Haworth Press, Inc.) Vol. 10, No. 3/4, 1998, pp. xiii-xvi; and: *New International Directions in HIV Prevention for Gay and Bisexual Men* (ed: Michael T. Wright, B. R. Simon Rosser, and Onno de Zwart) The Haworth Press, Inc., 1998, pp. xiii-xvi; and: *New International Directions in HIV Prevention for Gay and Bisexual Men* (ed: Michael T. Wright, B. R. Simon Rosser, and Onno de Zwart) Harrington Park Press, an imprint of The Haworth Press, Inc., 1998, pp. xiii-xvi. Single or multiple copies of this article are available for a fee from The Haworth Document Delivery Service [1-800-342-9678, 9:00 a.m. - 5:00 p.m. (EST). E-mail address: getinfo@haworthpressinc.com].

© 1998 by The Haworth Press, Inc. All rights reserved.

The symposia participants included both researchers and practitioners, representing a diversity of cultures, experiences, and disciplines:

Philippe Adam (France) of CNRS, Paris

Wayne Blankenship (USA), San Francisco AIDS Foundation

Michael Bochow (Germany), Intersofia, Berlin

Tom Coates (USA), Center for AIDS Prevention Studies (CAPS), University of California at San Francisco

Peter Davies (UK), Sigma Research, London

Onno de Zwart (Netherlands), Municipal Health Service Rotterdam Area

Peter Keogh (UK), Sigma Research, London

Rommel Mendès-Leite (France), The Laboratory of Social Anthropology (LAS-EHESS)/The Research Group for the Study of Sexuality (GREH), Paris

Dave Nimmons (USA), Gay Men's Health Crisis (GMHC), New York

Eric Rofes (USA), University of California at Berkeley, Graduate School of Education

Rolf Rosenbrock (Germany), Social Science Research Center Berlin (WZB)

B. R. Simon Rosser (USA), University of Minnesota Medical School, Department of Family Practice and Community Health

Marie-Ange Schiltz (France), CAMS–CNRS–EHESS, Paris

Matthias Weikert (Germany), The Department for Work, Health, and Social Welfare, Office of Health Promotion/AIDS, Hamburg

The articles assembled here reflect the depth and breadth of the topics discussed at the meetings. In preparing their chapters, each author was given the freedom to choose an issue which she or he felt was of central importance to the future of prevention. Each author was also able to choose a style appropriate to the information she or he wished to communicate. The result is a richly textured presentation of ideas incorporating both academic and journalistic elements, so as to reach a diverse audience and to promote reflection in all parts of the prevention community.

The unifying theme within this book is that of context. As became clear during the symposia, there is consensus among the authors that prevention theory and practice needs to move beyond a discussion of discreet risk behaviors to include consideration of the context in which men have sex with other men. The articles here suggest that this context includes such aspects as the nature of the sexual relationship, community opinion and norms, altruistic motivations, the special rationality of love, and the HIV status of the men involved. From many different perspectives, the writers argue that we have concentrated too much energy on campaigns which oversimplify sex between men. In the future we need to take into account the multi-layered and ultimately very individual way in which HIV-risk is managed. This will mean developing strategies which are more closely based on the everyday realities of men's sexual lives. In so doing, the authors contend, prevention will be more relevant and, hopefully, more effective.

The first two articles by Michael T. Wright serve as an introduction, providing an overview of major themes which are developed in more detail within the following chapters. The first chapter presents a joint statement of recommendations for the future of prevention which was produced at the first symposium. The second chapter presents a general critique of HIV prevention and research from the perspective of leading European theorists. Chapters 3 and 4, written by Marie-Ange Schiltz and Michael Bochow, respectively, present analyses of population-based data from France and Germany which illustrate complex trends that cannot be explained by using the typical slogans of prevention campaigns. Both articles illustrate the importance of including the influences of contextual factors, even when interpreting the quantitative data from large national samples.

The next two articles present aspects of the social context of HIV transmission. Peter Keogh and colleagues examine how prevention campaigns have ignored the different needs of HIV positive versus HIV negative men, reflecting how the issue of serostatus is a taboo within the gay community. David Nimmons looks at the issue of altruism, posing the hypothesis that men caring for one another is an important motivation for preventive behavior. He further discusses the ways in which AIDS has brought forth caring attitudes in men and asks the question why these attitudes have been so ignored in our prevention work.

In articles seven and eight, Onno de Zwart and colleagues as well as Rommel Mendès-Leite shed light on the personal context, discussing some of the mechanisms which bring meaning and structure to sexual relationships. de Zwart presents results of a qualitative study in the Netherlands which shows the complex meanings and situations connected with anal sex. In contrast to much HIV prevention material, which often depicts condom use as easy and matter-of-fact, the Dutch men interviewed reveal issues of trust, pleasure, and power which enter into their decisions to have anal sex. Mendès-Leite focuses on what he calls "imaginary protections," ways in which people subjectively appropriate HIV prevention messages so as to maximize their sexual needs being met. It is not that people ignore preventive measures, he argues, but it is the unique rationality of sexuality which allows for both risk-taking and the illusion of being safe from disease.

Articles nine and ten present broad critiques of prevention work in the U.S.A. within the larger societal and cultural context. Both Wayne Blankenship and Eric Rofes unite observations from gay culture and from the AIDS service movement to suggest changes which need to take place at a macro level in order for prevention to be more effective.

In the final two articles, B. R. Simon Rosser and Michael T. Wright discuss prevention in the context of the AIDS service movement. The first article addresses the issues raised by the new and more effective treatments which have become available. The second reports on meetings held two consecutive years at a national conference in the U.S.A. during which prevention providers identified a host of factors, both within and outside of the movement, which are changing prevention practice.

It is our sincere hope that the ideas contained in the following pages will stimulate readers to examine critically the practice of HIV prevention so as to be able to develop innovative approaches for meeting the challenges of the future.

Michael T. Wright, LICSW, MS
B. R. Simon Rosser, PhD, MPH
Onno de Zwart, MA

Acknowledgments

The symposia on which this collection of articles is based were organized and financed by the Deutsche AIDS-Hilfe, the national German AIDS organization. Additional support was provided by Pharmacia & Upjohn (USA). The authors would also like to thank all colleagues who attended the public discussions in Seattle, Vancouver, and Atlanta. Their comments and questions were important in shaping the contributions for this volume.

The Chorin Document: A Joint Statement of Recommendations for HIV Prevention Targeting Men Who Have Sex with Men

Michael T. Wright, LICSW, MS

SUMMARY. This article is a joint statement of recommendations for HIV prevention in industrialized countries targeting men who have sex with men. The statement was issued at an international symposium of HIV prevention practitioners and theorists organized in 1996 by the Deutsche AIDS-Hilfe, the national German AIDS organization. The objectives of the symposium were: (1) To identify and critically examine current paradigms; (2) To promote a deeper and more intensive debate; (3) To create a basis for new international collaborative ventures; and, (4) To consolidate and advance international discussion. The meeting focused on three topics: (1) New and neglected factors influencing people to engage in sexual acts which increase or decrease risk; (2) The meaning of sexuality/sexual acts and identity; and, (3) The factors fostering or impeding the implementation of prevention strategies, present and future. Among the recommendations made by the participants are: placing a greater focus on protective factors as opposed to risk factors; examining the meaning and context of sexual acts more closely; moving beyond prescriptive advice on sexual safety; and expanding beyond an ex-

[Haworth co-indexing entry note]: "The Chorin Document: A Joint Statement of Recommendations for HIV Prevention Targeting Men Who Have Sex with Men." Wright, Michael T. Co-published simultaneously in *Journal of Psychology & Human Sexuality* (The Haworth Press, Inc.) Vol. 10, No. 3/4, 1998, pp. 1-6; and: *New International Directions in HIV Prevention for Gay and Bisexual Men* (ed: Michael T. Wright, B. R. Simon Rosser, and Onno de Zwart) The Haworth Press, Inc., 1998, pp. 1-6; and: *New International Directions in HIV Prevention for Gay and Bisexual Men* (ed: Michael T. Wright, B. R. Simon Rosser, and Onno de Zwart) Harrington Park Press, an imprint of The Haworth Press, Inc., 1998, pp. 1-6. Single or multiple copies of this article are available for a fee from The Haworth Document Delivery Service [1-800-342-9678, 9:00 a.m. - 5:00 p.m. (EST). E-mail address: getinfo@haworthpressinc.com].

© 1998 by The Haworth Press, Inc. All rights reserved.

clusive focus on HIV so as to include other health issues. *[Article copies available for a fee from The Haworth Document Delivery Service: 1-800-342-9678. E-mail address: getinfo@haworthpressinc.com]*

Three symposia were organized in 1996 by the Deutsche AIDS-Hilfe, the national German AIDS organization, to stimulate an international discussion concerning the future of HIV prevention. These meetings not only resulted in the publication of this book, as described in the introduction, but also in the formulation of a unique joint statement concerning HIV prevention for gay and bisexual men. The document presented here was written during the first of the three symposia, held in Chorin, Germany. Included below are the names of the participants at the Chorin meeting and the full text of the recommendations given.

THE DOCUMENT

HIV prevention needs to change and be updated. What worked in the past will not necessarily work in the future. In order to develop new ways of reaching various populations so as to prevent the sexual transmission of this disease, the Deutsche AIDS-Hilfe, the national German AIDS organization, sponsored this international symposium.

The goals of this meeting were:

1. To identify and critically examine current paradigms;
2. To promote a deeper and more intensive debate;
3. To create a basis for new international collaborative ventures; and,
4. To consolidate and advance international discussion.

The objective of this meeting was to formulate recommendations for the future of primary prevention research and practice.

THE PARTICIPANTS

We, the participants of the symposium, represent a broad spectrum of expertise from four countries:

Wayne Blankenship, San Francisco AIDS Foundation, U.S.A.

Michael Bochow, Intersofia, Berlin, Germany.

Tom Coates, Center for AIDS Prevention Studies (CAPS), University of California at San Francisco, U.S.A.

Onno de Zwart, Municipal Health Service Rotterdam Area, The Netherlands.

Rommel Mendès-Leite, Laboratoire d'anthropologie sociale (LAS-EHESS)/Groupe de Recherches et d'Etudes sur l'Homosexualité et les sexualités (GREH), Paris, France.

Dave Nimmons, Gay Men's Health Crisis (GMHC), New York, U.S.A.

Eric Rofes, University of California at Berkeley, Graduate School of Education, San Francisco, U.S.A.

Rolf Rosenbrock, Social Science Research Center Berlin (WZB), Germany.

Marie-Ange Schiltz, CAMS–CNRS–EHESS, Paris, France.

Matthias Weikert, Freie und Hansestadt Hamburg Behörde für Arbeit, Gesundheit und Soziales, Gesundheitsförderung/AIDS, Hamburg, Germany.

Michael Wright, Deutsche AIDS-Hilfe, Berlin, Germany.

Early in the meeting we decided to set parameters for the discussion which both recognized the limited duration of the symposium and some of the important issues facing primary prevention today. The selected themes also reflect the areas in which we have the most knowledge and experience. We decided to speak from the context of the sexual transmission of HIV between men in Western industrialized countries where HIV is endemic. We agreed to consider three topics with respect to the ethnic, socioeconomic, developmental, experiential, and biographical diversity of men who have sexual contact with other men.

We focused on the following three topics:

1. New and neglected factors influencing people to engage in sexual acts which increase or decrease risk;
2. The meaning of sexuality/sexual acts and identity; and,
3. The factors fostering or impeding the implementation of prevention strategies, present and future.

In formulating our recommendations, we recognized not only similarities between our respective points of view, but also important differences of opinion concerning the primary prevention of HIV/AIDS. These differences reflect the diversity of disciplines, cultures, and experiences which we bring to our work. We found ourselves, at times, discussing fundamentally different perspectives, resulting in our not always being able to reach general consensus concerning our ideas for the future. Although each recommendation does not reflect the opinion of all participants, we, as a group, recommend using this document for a continued critical examination of our work and how we can develop our ideas to meet the evolving demands of preventing the spread of HIV/AIDS.

These recommendations, and the diversity of opinion which they represent, reflect important themes within the current debate. They also represent a challenge to us all to question the assumptions which we bring to our work and to go beyond generally accepted paradigms of research and practice.

NEW AND NEGLECTED FACTORS INFLUENCING PEOPLE TO ENGAGE IN SEXUAL ACTS WHICH INCREASE OR DECREASE RISK

In order to improve the efficacy of primary prevention, research and prevention practice must:

1. Focus on what keeps people safe and healthy instead of what places them at risk. We need to focus on what types of support, in what ways, and under what conditions men of any serostatus find strategies and draw on resources (material and immaterial, personal and social) to enhance and maintain safer behavior.
2. Include motivators broader than narrow self-interest; for example, altruism, the need for affiliation (with partners, networks, friends, communities), and the relationships and responsibilities within our partnerships and communities.
3. Admit that there will exist many questions for which simple prescriptive advice is not sufficient. Stimulating men's own discourse–both about HIV issues and larger psychosocial issues (e.g., life transition, intimacy, discrimination)–is a valuable end in itself within our communities. Our goal is to support men in engaging their own processes and clarifying their own values in deciding what is right for them. The attempt to exclude ambiguity and complexity from prevention has not proved helpful.
4. As early as possible, support younger gay men in identifying not only risks for HIV, but also resources and values which they can use

to stay uninfected. These resources should include the experiences of men who have stayed uninfected for many years.
5. More fully elucidate and address the role of both legal and illegal psychoactive substances in determining safer behavior.

THE MEANING OF SEXUALITY/SEXUAL ACTS AND IDENTITY

1. Research is needed concerning the following questions: Is it possible to comprehend, utilize, and accelerate shifts in meanings regarding specific sex acts in specific social groups? If so, how and over what time periods? To answer these questions, we suggest beginning qualitative research of cohorts, following different groups of gay men through the trajectories of their sexuality and identity.
2. Researchers must explain, richly and in detail, why they use specific sexual language in surveys and/or allow subjects themselves to determine the terms used in the research describing men's sexuality.
3. HIV prevention workers must acknowledge that sex acts are not discrete, mechanistic behaviors but are rich in diverse meanings and are constituted in a complex social and cultural context. We must challenge prevention work which treats acts as unimportant, interchangeable, or easily adaptable.
4. Prevention might aim to provide spaces where men can talk with one another about the meanings, feelings, realities, and fantasies of specific sexual acts. We might do this in various forms: support groups, street outreach, media debates, etc. We also need to develop new, diverse strategies, based on the structures of existing social groups.
5. We must take seriously the different forms of rational thought and logic which men use to explain and make sense of their sexual behavior. This is the starting point for working with men who have sex with men. It is important not to devalue the various ways men describe their sexuality by characterizing certain explanations as being excuses or the result of irrational thinking. It is also necessary to integrate specific sexual subcultures (non-monogamy, sadomasochism, etc.) into prevention and to accept these subcultures as social realities, fully valuing the associated practices and ways of life. HIV prevention practice needs to be adapted to the diversity of these subcultures.
6. HIV prevention must consider that specific acts are constituted out of gender-based identities. For example, penetration is often closely intertwined with male identities.

THE FACTORS FOSTERING OR IMPEDING THE IMPLEMENTATION OF HIV PREVENTION STRATEGIES, PRESENT AND FUTURE

1. HIV prevention programs should empower individuals to take responsibility for decisions around sexual risks and to accept the diversity of various lifestyles (i.e., bisexuals, men in primary relationships, etc.). It is important to:

   - Stress the skills of decision-making and negotiation for younger men; and,
   - Validate successful personal strategies over time for adult men/older men.

2. New opportunities for gay socialization must be created to expand individual options beyond activities which have to do with sex, HIV, and a narrow conception of sexual identity. For some individuals this may mean strengthening their identity within their own non-gay neighborhoods or ethnic communities.

3. We need to develop cooperation between organizations in industrialized countries where lifestyles of gay/bisexual men are similar. The purpose of working together would be:

   - Sharing successes, failures, and difficulties;
   - Understanding the range of prevention elsewhere so as to better design specific local programs; and,
   - Using our collective power to ensure adequate standards of civil rights and prevention funding.

4. Gay men's lives and their contributions to society must be acknowledged by the general population through each country's ensuring civil rights, legalization of partnerships, and adequate funding for services.

5. Public education should include non-judgmental information about sexual diversity and information about HIV prevention for sexually active youth.

6. HIV prevention strategies for the future will need to expand beyond the current focus. HIV prevention may shift from concentrating on HIV exclusively to including new issues and new allies. We must develop new programs for those affected by the multiple oppression of poverty and racism. We must empower ourselves to experiment and be creative, without always demanding quantifiable proof of our success.

Beyond Risk Factors:
Trends in European Safer Sex Research

Michael T. Wright, LICSW, MS

SUMMARY. This article provides an overview of important themes in European research regarding sexual behavior and the risk for HIV infection. There is a growing critique of HIV prevention among European theorists which focuses on four themes: (1) That current models over-emphasize the role of rational decision-making in sexual behavior; (2) That the individual is viewed as the unit of research and intervention; (3) That the person is assumed to be static, having qualities which remain unchanged over time; and, (4) That the social/cultural context of human interaction is ignored in relation to sexual behavior. To counteract these perceived deficiencies, it is proposed that future research and practice incorporate the following elements: sexual behavior as being primarily an interaction between persons as opposed to a decision of individuals; the effects of time on sexual decision-making; the cultural context and its influence on sexuality; the subjective experience of love as relates to sex; the role of power in determining sexual interaction; and the symbolic meaning of sexual acts. *[Article copies available for a fee from The Haworth Document Delivery Service: 1-800-342-9678. E-mail address: getinfo@haworthpressinc.com]*

The pursuit of dangerous sex is not as simple as mere thrill-seeking, or self-destructiveness. It may represent deep and mostly unconscious thinking about desire and the conditions that make life worthwhile. (Warner 1995, p. 35)

It was not dark, they were not drunk, and they did know what they were doing. (A maxim of Peter Davies, British sociologist.)

Now well into the second decade of the AIDS pandemic, the question of why people take the risk of becoming infected with HIV when having sex has become a topic of intense study and growing debate. The earliest researchers defined the language and parameters of the discussion, introducing such concepts as the Health Belief Model, risk factors, safe and unsafe sex, and relapse. Studies have focused on the individuals who are having unprotected intercourse in an attempt to define those qualities which lead to putting oneself at risk (Hospers & Kok, 1995). Such factors as low self-esteem, drug and alcohol use, and believing in one's own invulnerability have been supported in many investigations. However, there is a growing critique of these early studies. Leading the debate are a number of European investigators, many of whom have not published in English, or whose work predominantly appears in another language (e.g., Martin Dannecker, Michael Bochow, Michael Pollack, Marie-Ange Schiltz). The work of these researchers challenges some fundamental assumptions in HIV/AIDS prevention, particularly as found in the United States. In order to promote international discussion of these issues, this article provides an overview of the critique aimed at the earlier studies and of the major themes found in the current work of leading European investigators.

A EUROPEAN CRITIQUE OF SAFER SEX RESEARCH

The German researcher Rolf Rosenbrock (1995) summarizes the fundamental argument forming the basis of the European critique of the current safer sex debate. Rosenbrock identifies the early focus on risk factors as being a fundamental problem in the literature. According to his analysis, the risk factor discussion is based largely on the assumption that human sexuality can be divided into discrete behaviors which are under the control of the individual. Social Learning (e.g., Bandura and the Health Belief Model) and related theories–focusing on the individual's ability to make reasoned decisions regarding his/her health when provided with adequate information–formed an important theoretical foundation for the development of this assumption. The resultant idea that sexual behavior is subject primarily to the reasoning capacities of the individual has led to a reductionism which ignores the depth and complexity of the human sexual experience. He and others are calling for an expansion of the parameters of the research so as to take into account the broader realities. Peter Aggleton

(1995) of the World Health Organization articulates this view in appealing for a shift from the acquisition and practice of knowledge and behaviors to an examination of their context and consequences. This means focusing on how sexuality is understood and lived as opposed to what individuals know and do. According to Aggleton, today's population-based surveys provide inadequate information as to the context in which sex occurs (see also Cohen, 1995a; Montgomery et al., 1989; Pollack & Moatti, 1990).

Essentially, the sources consulted for this article are proposing an expansion of the current paradigm. The basic scientific validity and relevance of the bulk of safer sex research is not being called into question. Rather, they are advocating for an extension of the current analysis so as to include neglected elements of human sexuality in relation to HIV/AIDS. Figure 1, inspired by Guizzardi (1995), offers a simple, elucidating image which depicts this goal.

As a result of reducing human sexuality to a small number of behaviors and measurable elements, researchers have run the risk of pathologizing normal behavior. According to Vincke (1995), there is an increasing moralizing quality in research hypotheses which can be summarized in the statement: Why are they still having unsafe sex? Such hypotheses imply that *they* should know better. Many Europeans (e.g., Davies et al., 1993; Mendès-Leite, 1995) are of the view that, to date, research has largely

FIGURE 1. Expanding the Paradigm in Safer Sex Research

Time	Culture	International Perspective
Current Theory and Practice		Symbolic Meaning
Risk Factors: self-esteem, alcohol/drug use, feelings of invulnerability, other psychological factors		
Individuals as Unit of Research/Intervention		Power
Rational Decision Making		
		Love

overlooked the normal and complex human elements of sexual behavior which lead to unprotected sex: for example, the increased pleasure experienced by many people when not using a condom and the problems inherent in thinking about sexuality as a conditioned behavior (Bochow, 1995a, b). Further, this pathologizing of normal sexual acts can lead to intense feelings of shame and guilt when one has unprotected sex, making it that much more difficult to have an open dialogue with one's partners and social network about one's questions and concerns regarding safer sex.

A major impetus for this developing critique of established theories of safer sex research has come from qualitative studies of gay men who are having unprotected intercourse. The data have led theorists to believe that, beyond the commonly discussed *risk factors*, there are many other subjective reasons and processes which result in unsafe sex. These involve such common experiences as love, intimacy, and the meaning of sexuality in people's lives. This growing body of information is casting doubt on the idea that certain individuals are at risk of HIV infection. By virtue of our humanity, we are all potentially capable of having unsafe sex, given the right set of circumstances. This insight prompts us to broaden the focus of safer sex research methodology and prevention efforts.

The critique of the dominant trends in safer sex research to date can be described in more detail by discussing four major themes which occur among the various theorists:

1. That current models over-emphasize the role of rational decision-making in sexual behavior;
2. That the individual is viewed as the unit of research and intervention;
3. That the person is assumed to be static, having qualities which remain unchanged over time; and,
4. That the social/cultural context of human interaction is ignored in relation to sexual behavior.

Rational Decision Making. The assumption that sex is a rational process can be questioned. When one is wanting to have sex, the ability to make reasoned decisions is only *one* of various influences on a person's behavior, and often not the primary one. Therefore, providing information, even in the most accessible and attractive form, does not ensure follow-through in terms of condom use. There is not a clear, linear causal chain of events between learning that a sexual activity is potentially dangerous and deciding whether or not to perform this behavior. What one does is a product of causal chains which involve various elements, both interactional and nonrational (Ahlemeyer, 1995).

The Individual As Unit of Research and Intervention. Individuals do not make the decision alone whether or not to perform a certain sexual act. Each person decides in relation to his or her partner(s). Unprotected sex results from the communication of a dyad which builds upon, but is not determined by, the knowledge base of the individual (Ahlemeyer, 1995; Sandfort, 1995). Therefore, each sexual act must be seen as the product of a dyad, and partnering as the appropriate level for intervention. Sexual behavior is a negotiation between two people in the context of their relationship (Ahlemeyer, 1995; Bochow, 1995a; Guizzardi, 1995). This critique is supported by the large number of studies which show that unprotected anal intercourse among gay men is most likely to occur within established partnerships (Bochow, 1995a; Coxon, 1995; Hospers & Kok, 1995; Martin et al., 1989; Vincke, 1995).

The Person As Static Entity. Many research studies concerning HIV and safer sex assume that qualities of individuals which are measured (e.g., self-esteem) are fixed personal traits which have to do primarily with the person him/herself. These traits can in turn be used to predict behavior. This assumption ignores the strong influence of context. Certain locations, certain people, certain relationships, certain events, etc., may evoke different feelings and thoughts, leading to very different reactions and behaviors. Also, the timing of certain events or encounters can play an important role in how they are perceived (Cohen, 1995b; Ingham, 1995). To quote a maxim of the British researcher, Peter Davies, "In the end, we all relapse" (Davies et al., 1992), meaning that given the complex nature of human sexuality, all of us could find ourselves in a set of circumstances under which we would be likely to have unprotected sex.

The Social Context of Sexual Interaction. The social context of sex is ignored by many researchers. Culture plays a crucial role in determining how sexuality is defined and experienced and whether certain behaviors (e.g., using a condom or taking an active role in negotiating sexual behavior) are permissible and under what circumstances (Cohen, 1995b; Guizzardi, 1995; Ingham, 1995). Culture also determines the relative value of our actions and the roles we play. For example, it may be more important for a woman to remain passive within a sexual relationship and thereby allow unsafe sex than to assume an assertive role by insisting on condom use (Cohen, 1995b).

EXPANDING THE HORIZONS OF FUTURE RESEARCH

European investigators not only offer a critique of the dominant theories to date, but also propose their own concepts toward expanding the theoretical basis of safer sex research. Their ideas can be organized under six headings: the interactional perspective; time; culture; love; power; and symbolic meaning.

1. The Interactional Perspective. European HIV prevention researchers have begun concentrating on the nature of sexual partnerships (Bochow, 1995a; Hubert, 1995). What is it within the communication of partners which leads to various sexual behaviors? How is sex negotiated and what are the elements of this negotiation? What is intimacy and how is it expressed sexually? A number of theorists claim that we have overlooked the very reason for coupling, namely to be intimate with another person, and how a couple functions in order to build and maintain their union to one another (Dannecker, 1994; Davies et al., 1993; Prieur, 1991). This function can conceivably take precedent over other needs, such as to protect each other from HIV (Bochow, 1995b). In fact, the act of using a condom can itself be seen as preventing the closeness that is desired (Henriksson, 1995; Prieur, 1991). By including the role of the partner-dyad in sexual interactions, the focus on the individual is complemented and expanded to account for the effects of relationship on sexual decision-making.

2. Time. To address what has been criticized as being the static nature of investigations in this area, many theorists are looking to the concepts of time and situation, studying the location and timing of sexual behavior. This includes finding out about what other needs a person has and what priority these needs have in relation to safer sex. Cohen (1995b) provides this example: If a person is in great financial need to support his/her family and there is a lucrative opportunity for prostitution, with more money being offered if s/he is willing to forego using a condom, the need for income can supersede the need for risk-avoidance. This example also illustrates the aspect of time, in that an intangible future (having a longer life without HIV) may not be not as important as today's concrete basic needs. Time also plays a role when, in the development of a relationship, sex is being negotiated, when in the person's own developmental process s/he is having sex, and at what stage in the epidemic the person is having the sexual contact (Cohen, 1995b; Ingham, 1995). Therefore the factors of time and situation potentially influence a person's response at any given moment, making such traits as fear, anxiety, self-esteem, and vulnerability relative and changeable.

3. Culture. Culture is also important in the determination of sexual behavior regarding HIV risk. Calvez (1995) notes that different cultures view risk differently; certain cultural settings require people to take risks in order to prove their loyalty and commitment to the larger group. Therefore, although the person knows s/he is taking a risk of contracting HIV, it may be more important in terms of being part of the larger group to have sex without using a condom. Calvez gives the example of gay farmers in Brittany. There one finds a culture of autonomy and independence which supports an attitude rejecting the use of condoms; to use a condom would be to lose status among peers. Cohen (1995b) provides another example from cultures he has encountered in his work in developing countries. Among some peoples, the exchange of semen is identified explicitly as being a sign of closeness and love. This message runs counter to safer sex guidelines. The culture, forming the basis of human interaction in the society, takes precedent, resulting in few members using condoms. Beyond peer norms, deeper cultural and societal influences which determine the primary identities and roles of people can work in complex ways to determine whether or not one performs protected sex.

4. *Love.* The non-quantifiable romantic dimensions of sexuality are also overlooked in thinking of sex as being definable in terms of discrete behaviors. Love, pleasure, and desire are expressed in the common everyday language of relationships and sexual intimacy, but are largely ignored in HIV prevention research (Prieur, 1995). Within the German literature, one finds reference to the *risk factor love*, an intentionally ironic label for the elements of an encounter which make one fall in love with another person and want to trust him/her. These elements need more attention, particularly as they are played out in the dyad of a sexual relationship. By including this dimension of sexuality, researchers can begin acknowledging those very human, albeit difficult to quantify, experiences during which we choose to give ourselves over to another person.

5. *Power.* Power plays an important role, not only within the dyad of sexual partners, but also within the society at large, in determining sexual roles and behaviors. Power is played out in terms of control and surrender within the sexual encounter. Whether one seeks to control or surrender is determined by many factors, including culture, gender, role in society, and subcultural norms (de Zwart, 1995; Prieur, 1994). HIV has resulted in a unique challenge to this dynamic, introducing the element of protection. The problem is that this element can be experienced as anathema to both the experiences of conquest and being taken. Without surrender and control, sexuality can lose its deeper meanings and therefore its physical and emotional satisfaction for partners. Given the choice between dissatisfying protected sex, and satisfying unprotected sex, many would choose the latter, responding to a very basic need (de Zwart, 1995; Prieur, 1991). Research needs to pay attention to finding out more about this sexual dynamic and how safer sex may play a role.

6. Symbolic Meaning. Sexual behavior can be seen as functioning under its own rationality. The problem with focusing on rationality in the conventional sense (logical decisions based on knowledge) is that this special form of rationality is ignored (Mendès-Leite, 1995). Sexual decision-making only partly involves conventional reason. In addition to factual information, the person calls upon deep-lying and often unconscious symbolic meanings which influence his/her behavior. Regarding HIV, the knowledge level can give messages saying that unprotected anal sex is dangerous, while the symbolic level generates images of sex without a condom in response to a deep need, such as intimacy. There can also be profound symbolic associations with specific acts, such as ingesting semen, which are experienced as integral to one's sexual life (Prieur, 1991). According to Mendès-Leite (1995), the interaction of the symbolic and knowledge-based levels can produce a filtering process which results in the construction of "imaginary protections." The person engages in self-deception in order to get the symbolic needs met. Once s/he finds the ideal person to have unprotected sex with, s/he constructs criteria to convince him/herself that this partner is not infected. This process is not to be viewed as pathological, but as a normal response of a person finding a way around the epidemic in order to meet deeply felt needs which can only be expressed symbolically, (for example, the need to have contact with semen or the need to have anal sex (Henriksson, 1995)).

IMPLICATIONS OF AN EXPANDED PARADIGM

In incorporating the above critique within the current theory and practice of safer sex research and HIV prevention work, new possibilities arise. In the attempt to gain more in-depth information about people's experience of protected and unprotected sex, we can begin to routinely supplement current empirical work with qualitative studies designed to expand our ability to more creatively interpret the data we are collecting. This can include incorporating more qualitative elements within our research designs as well as expanding the role of focus groups and other means of dialogue in evaluating our prevention efforts. And instead of using the resultant input to buttress current models, we can challenge ourselves to look for keys to a new paradigm to use in our work.

In our prevention campaigns, there is the opportunity for a more honest and open discussion about current sexual behavior, avoiding potentially pejorative labels such as "relapse" and working outside models of norm reinforcement. As reported in the *Journal du Sida* (Elovich, 1995), GMHC (Gay Men's Health Crisis) in New York has begun incorporating a model for discussion in which no themes are treated as taboo. Actively promoting a norm of safer sex takes a back seat to promoting a new level of dialogue regarding the meanings of sexual behavior. The information and experience thus gained will prepare us for the development of the next phase of prevention initiatives.

We are also invited to examine our choice of words when talking about sexuality and HIV/AIDS. Are there alternatives to the terms "relapse" and "recidivism," whose origins are in the fields of epidemiology, substance abuse, and criminology? Even terms such as "safe" and "unsafe" may need to be replaced with such descriptors as "protected" and "unprotected" so as not to confuse the decision-making process with connotations of failure or pathology.

Our sensitivity to multiculturalism can be heightened by allowing cultural factors to play an increasing role in our analysis and practice. Although current models, particularly as found in the United States, have made serious efforts to incorporate cultural differences in designing and implementing HIV prevention programs, perhaps we can expand our thinking further to consider more specifically the ways in which culture can supersede other factors in determining the sexual behavior of people. And perhaps we can allow the perspectives of various cultures to more dramatically affect the formulation and application of new paradigms for our work.

Also, we have the possibility of lifting the burden from individuals, especially those in the most affected groups, who are already faced with the problem of discrimination at the personal and societal levels. Moving from a deficit-based model to a more complex view of human sexuality, we can relieve the shame and guilt often experienced by people when they engage in risky behavior. The individual can thus be invited to stop thinking of safer sex in terms of personal success and failure and to instead enter a dialogue in which s/he can consider the meanings which (unprotected) sex has in his/her life.

We can build on the sex-positive perspective which we have promoted in safer sex research and education. We can take as a starting point that sex without a condom is a normal human behavior in response to a profound need for intimacy with other people. Thus avoiding the pathologizing of certain sexual acts, we can create a more open climate for both researcher and subject, client and worker to talk about what really happens in those most intimate moments between two human beings.

There is also the possibility of moving from a risk-elimination to a harm-reduction perspective which respects individuals' and couples' risk-taking within their sexual lives. This perspective recognizes the ability of people to consider risk and to incorporate it into their decision-making process, while at the same time acknowledging that risk-taking is also a normal part of everyday life.

Finally, we are at the brink of a new phase in sexual research in which the symbolic meaning of human sexuality can be recognized in all its complexity and apparent contradiction. The meaning of being entered in intercourse, of touching a partner's semen, of experiencing abandon within a human relationship can have profound effects on the person which have to do with the meaning of life itself. The world's art and literature attest to these meanings and to the intricate relationship between death and sexuality. We can begin now to allow these insights to affect our theoretical and practical work in HIV/AIDS prevention.

CONCLUSION

AIDS work has always been the work of pioneers. Within the social sciences, research regarding safer sex has provided unique challenges. We have been confronted with both the greatest success in the history of public health and with some of the most disturbing questions in attempting to understand and combat the spread of this serious epidemic. The challenge now is to continue in the spirit of breaking new ground, opening ourselves to the tremendous lessons HIV/AIDS has to teach us by not shying away from recognizing human sexuality in all of its mystery and contradiction. The growing critique from Europe is an ideal opportunity to expand the theoretical basis of the work done to date so as to achieve new levels of efficacy in the struggle for health and human dignity.

REFERENCES

Aggleton, P. (1995). Priorities for social and behavioural research on HIV and AIDS. *AIDS in Europe-The Behavioural Aspect (Edition Sigma)*, Berlin, Germany. *1*:55-65.

Ahlemeyer, H. (1995). Heterosexual behaviour and AIDS prevention: The impact of intimate communication. *AIDS in Europe-The Behavioural Aspect (Edition Sigma)*, Berlin, Germany. *4*:17-27.

Bochow, M. (1995a). Datenwüsten und Deutungsarmut: Zu Defiziten in der Präventionsorientierten AIDS-Forschung am Beispiel der Zielgruppe homosexueller Männer. *Zeitschrift für Sexualforschung*, 39-48.

Bochow, M. (1995b). Je crois beaucoup à la notion de protection négociée. *Le Journal du Sida*, *72*:24-25.

Calvez, M. (1995). Perception of risks and commitment to a community: A cultural approach. *AIDS in Europe-The Behavioural Aspect (Edition Sigma), Berlin, Germany.* 4:39-49.

Cohen, M. (1995a). The health belief model: Always, sometimes, or never useful in guiding HIV/AIDS prevention. *AIDS in Europe-The Behavioural Aspect (Edition Sigma), Berlin, Germany.* 4:49-55.

Cohen, M. (1995b). The place of time in understanding sexual behaviour and risk of HIV infection. *AIDS in Europe-The Behavioural Aspect (Edition Sigma), Berlin, Germany.* 4:27-33.

Coxon, A. (1995). Change in gay men's risk behaviour: Relapse or rationality– One, both or neither? *AIDS in Europe-The Behavioural Aspect (Edition Sigma), Berlin, Germany.* 2:133-147.

Dannecker, M. (1994). Im Liebesfall. *Aktuell-Das Magazin der Deutschen AIDS-Hilfe.* 7:16-20.

Davies, P. et al. (1992). On relapse: Recidivism or rational response? In P. Aggleton et al., *AIDS: Rights, Risks and Reason.* London.

Davies, P. et al. (1993). *Sex, Gay Men and AIDS.* London: Falmer Press.

de Zwart, O. (1995). The structure and meaning of anal sex among gay men. *AIDS in Europe-The Behavioural Aspect (Edition Sigma), Berlin, Germany.* 2:107-115.

Elovich, R. (1995). L'important n'est pas de dire aux gays ce qu'ils doivent faire mais de les entendre dire ce qu'ils font. *Le Journal du Sida.* 72:28-29.

Guizzardi, G. (1995). Health belief model–Critiques and alternatives: The social discourse on AIDS. *AIDS in Europe-The Behavioural Aspect (Edition Sigma), Berlin, Germany.* 4:33-39.

Henriksson, B. (1995). Risk factor love: The symbolic meaning of sexuality and HIV prevention. *AIDS in Europe-The Behavioural Aspect (Edition Sigma), Berlin, Germany.* 2:115-133.

Hospers, H.J. & Kok, G. (1995). Determinants of safe and risk-taking behavior among gay men: A review. *AIDS Education and Prevention,* 7(1), pp. 74-96.

Hubert, M. (1995). Studying sexual behaviour and HIV risk: Towards a pan-European approach. *AIDS in Europe-The Behavioural Aspect (Edition Sigma), Berlin, Germany.* 1:65-75.

Ingham, R. (1995). Towards an alternative model of sexual behaviour. *AIDS in Europe-The Behavioural Aspect (Edition Sigma), Berlin, Germany.* 4:15-17.

Kippax, S., Dowsett, G., Davis, M., Rodden, P., & Crawford, J. (1993). *Sustaining Safe Sex: Gay Communities Respond to AIDS.* London: Falmer Press.

Martin, J., Dean, L., Garcia, M., & Hall, W. (1989). The impact of AIDS on a gay community: Changes in sexual behavior, substance use, and mental health. *American Journal of Community Psychology,* 17(3):269-293.

Mendès-Leite, R. (1995). The meaning of otherness: Male homosexualities and "imaginary protections." *AIDS in Europe-The Behavioural Aspect (Edition Sigma), Berlin, Germany.* 2:97-107.

Montgomery, S., Joseph, J., Becker, M., Ostrow, D., Kessler, R., & Kirscht, P. (1989). The health belief model in understanding compliance with preventive recommendation for AIDS: How useful? *AIDS Education and Prevention, 1*:303-323.

Pollack, M. & Moatti J.-P. (1990). HIV risk perception and determinants of sexual behaviour. In M. Hubert (ed.). *Sexual Behaviour and Risks of HIV Infection: Proceedings of an International Workshop Supported by the European Communities.* Brussels: Publication des Facultés Universitaires Saint-Louis, 17-38.

Prieur, A. (1990). Norwegian gay men: Reasons for continued practice of unsafe sex. *AIDS Education and Prevention, 2*(2):109-115.

Prieur, A. (1991). Mann-Männliche Liebe in den Zeiten von AIDS: eine Untersuchung zum Sexualverhalten norwegischer homosexueller Männer. Deutsche AIDS-Hilfe, Berlin.

Prieur, A. (1994). "I am my own special creation": Mexican homosexual transvestites' construction of femininity. *Young, Nordic Journal of Youth Research, 2*:2.

Prieur, A. (1995). Sexual negotiations and symbolic dimensions: Introduction. *AIDS in Europe–The Behavioural Aspect (Edition Sigma), Berlin, Germany.* 2:95-97.

Rosenbrock, R. (1995). Social sciences and HIV/AIDS policies: Experiences and perspectives. *AIDS in Europe–The Behavioural Aspect (Edition Sigma), Berlin, Germany.* 1:259-273.

Sandfort, T. (1995). Does coping with HIV-infection affect safer sexual behaviour? *AIDS in Europe–The Behavioural Aspect (Edition Sigma), Berlin, Germany.* 2:101-193.

Vincke, J. (1995). The taboo: Sexual risk behaviour among people with HIV/AIDS: Introductory remarks. *AIDS in Europe–The Behavioural Aspect (Edition Sigma), Berlin, Germany.* 2:169-171.

Warner, M. (1995, January 31). Why gay men are having risky sex. *The Village Voice, XL*(5):32ff.

Not All Men, Situations, and Actions Are Equal: Moving from 100% Protection to a More Realistic Prevention Practice

Marie-Ange Schiltz, MA

SUMMARY. Since 1985, annual surveys conducted in the French gay press show that gay men in France have made considerable changes in their sexual behavior due to the AIDS epidemic. However, risky behavior still occurs. In this article, some ideas which have been assumed concerning residual risk among gay men are tested. The research questions were: (1) Should all unprotected acts of anal intercourse be considered risky? (2) Has a phenomenon of relapse really occurred among gay men in France? and, (3) Are risks only limited to men who are on the margin of the gay community? Before answering these questions, major landmarks in HIV prevention for gay men in France are reviewed. Then, on the basis of the results of the 1995 Gay Press Survey, subjects' perception of the degree to which they are socially accepted, and the diversity of homosexual lifestyles are presented. Finally, we describe how respondents have adjusted to HIV-risk at a time when there has been much talk about the re-emergence of risky behaviors and a resurgence of the AIDS epidemic among homosexual men. *[Article copies available for a fee from The Haworth Document Delivery Service: 1-800-342-9678. E-mail address: getinfo@haworthpressinc.com]*

[Haworth co-indexing entry note]: "Not All Men, Situations, and Actions Are Equal: Moving from 100% Protection to a More Realistic Prevention Practice." Schiltz, Marie-Ange. Co-published simultaneously in *Journal of Psychology & Human Sexuality* (The Haworth Press, Inc.) Vol. 10, No. 3/4, 1998, pp. 19-35; and: *New International Directions in HIV Prevention for Gay and Bisexual Men* (ed: Michael T. Wright, B. R. Simon Rosser, and Onno de Zwart) The Haworth Press, Inc., 1998, pp. 19-35; and: *New International Directions in HIV Prevention for Gay and Bisexual Men* (ed: Michael T. Wright, B. R. Simon Rosser, and Onno de Zwart) Harrington Park Press, an imprint of The Haworth Press, Inc., 1998, pp. 19-35. Single or multiple copies of this article are available for a fee from The Haworth Document Delivery Service [1-800-342-9678, 9:00 a.m. - 5:00 p.m. (EST). E-mail address: getinfo@haworthpressinc.com].

© 1998 by The Haworth Press, Inc. All rights reserved.

In line with research conducted in other countries during the 1970s which began studying homosexuality as a way of life (Bell & Weinberg, 1978; Dannecker & Reiche, 1974; Gagnon, 1973), Michael Pollak (1982) described the new *ghetto of organized cruising* which had arisen in France. This was at a time when the original gay political movement was in decline, while the gay-identified commercial sector was expanding. Pollak focused on how homosexual men sought to *rationally organize their sexuality* (Béjin & Pollak, 1977) by adopting a *lifestyle* meant to maximize pleasure and to minimize the emotional and social *consequences* ensuing from their sexual activities. In 1985, Pollak expanded his analysis to include quantitative population-based data on gay men in France. Beyond the lifestyle in the *ghetto*, Pollak (1982) examined the diversity and organization of the various homosexual ways of life among French men in general. With the advent of AIDS, Pollak argued that homosexual men had developed new approaches to how they organized their lives (Pollak, Schiltz & Laurindo, 1986). The previous work concerning homosexual lifestyle would serve as a basis for understanding how individuals managed the new risk of being infected with HIV. Since 1985, yearly surveys have continued to be conducted in the French gay press in order to measure over time the extent of safer sex practices among homosexual men.

We have noted that, for many years now, gays in France have made considerable changes in their sexual behavior due to the AIDS epidemic. However, risky behavior still occurs. In the data presented here, we tested some ideas which have been taken-for-granted concerning *residual risk* among gay men. Our research questions were: (1) Should all unprotected acts of anal intercourse be considered risky? (2) Has a phenomenon of *relapse* really occurred among gay men in France? and, (3) Are risks only limited to men who are not integrated into the community (often referred to as *men who have sex with men* in the American literature)?

Before answering these questions, we would like to present major landmarks in HIV prevention for gays in France. Then, on the basis of the results of the 1995 *Enquête Presse Gaie* (Gay Press Survey or GPS), we shall present our sampling procedure and methodology, the subjects' perception of the degree to which they are socially accepted, and the diversity of homosexual lifestyles represented in the sample. Finally, we will describe how respondents have adjusted to HIV-risk at a time when there has been much talk about the re-emergence of risky behaviors and a resurgence of the AIDS epidemic among homosexual men.

HIV PREVENTION LANDMARKS IN FRANCE

The first AIDS cases in France were diagnosed in the early eighties. In the initial years of the epidemic, surveillance data revealed that infections in France, as in other industrialized countries, were mainly among young homosexual men and intravenous drug users who were henceforth identified as *groups at risk*. The viral nature of the disease and the fact that it is sexually transmitted were established in 1983 (Montangier et al., 1983). The first French AIDS service organizations came into being at this time. Gay organizations and the gay press began to make HIV prevention recommendations to the gay population in 1984. The prevention model at the time promoted a risk-free sexual lifestyle with an emphasis on safe sex, which consisted of avoiding any exchange of body fluids (i.e., through systematic protection or abstinence from risk behaviors). To these messages was added the admonition to exercise more care when having sex, changing one's lifestyle by limiting one's exposure to HIV risk (e.g., by having fewer partners) and by removing oneself from the usual sexual networks.

In 1987, the AIDS service organizations' pioneering work was amplified by national public prevention campaigns and by the official authorization finally being granted to advertise condoms. A specific government-sponsored advertising campaign targeted at gays was initiated in the early nineties; a risk reduction or safer sex model replaced the no-risk message; and making condoms readily available became a priority of prevention for the gay population.

AWARENESS OF THE SCOPE OF THE EPIDEMIC AMONG FRENCH HOMOSEXUAL MEN

In 1985, homosexual men accounted for two-thirds of all recorded AIDS cases in France (World Health Organization, 1985). Although this figure had fallen significantly by 1996 (Lot, Pillonel, Pinget, Cazein, Gouzel & Laporte, 1997), homosexual men still accounted for 37% of the cases reported that year, making up the largest group in France infected by HIV (Réseau National de Santé Publique, 1997). The epidemic among gay men is highly concentrated in the capital: Paris and its region account for just under 50% of the cumulative AIDS cases in this transmission group since the start of the epidemic in France (Réseau National de Santé Publique, 1997).

It is also important to note that French homosexual men availed themselves of the HIV test quite early on (Schiltz & Adam, 1996); 32% of the respondents to our national survey had been tested as early as 1986. This rate came close to 90% in 1995. In our survey samples, the rate of positive results peaked at 22% in 1986 and has decreased from then on (Pollak and Schiltz, 1990). In 1995, 15% of the respondents tested were HIV-positive (Schiltz, 1997). Gay men thus found out quite early in the epidemic that their sexual networks in particular were significantly affected by HIV, confronting them directly with the necessity of prevention.

METHODS

Procedure. It is never easy to study a minority whose signs of group affiliation are not visible. According to several surveys in France and other industrialized countries, 4% of men have had sexual intercourse with other men and 1% during the past year (Messiah & Mouret-Fourme, 1995). To study the French gay population, we developed a four-page questionnaire which readers of gay newspapers and magazines are asked to send back. This survey has been inserted in major gay periodicals once a year since 1985. According to Michael Pollak (1981), a quantitative study can help us focus on the "banality of the facts" of homosexuality.

The present analysis is based on the last completed survey concerning the lifestyles of French gay men and the way they adjust to HIV risks. A self-administered questionnaire was inserted in ten French gay magazines in 1995. The total number of respondents was 2,616.

Subjects. In the sample, the men were better educated and were more likely to be from the middle class, as compared to single men in the French national census or in the large national survey on sexual behavior in France (ACSF: Analyse des comportements sexuels en France); the latter was conducted on a representative sample of 20,000 people between the ages of 18 and 69 in 1992 (Spira et al., 1994). Teenagers, retirees and, to a lesser extent, the jobless were underrepresented in our sample. The distribution method for the questionnaire as well as the self-selected nature of the sample are unique, as compared to other French sexual surveys. In comparison to gays in the ACSF, those who responded to the Gay Press Survey were more likely to be living in a couple with another man, while bisexuals in the two studies hardly differed in terms of partnership (Messiah & Mouret-Fourme, 1995). However, as we shall see in greater detail to follow, the number of partners reported by self-selected subjects, such as the respondents of the Gay Press Survey, is always higher than those reported in random samples, regardless of the type of sexual activity. Thus, our survey primarily includes men who openly acknowledge their homosexuality in their daily life and who actively engage in *cruising* (actively seeking male sex partners).

Although sexually active men (2% of GPS respondents had not had sexual intercourse during the preceding year compared with 6% of the men in the ACSF survey) and those who identified themselves as homosexual (87%) were overrepresented, the 1995 GPS sample is not composed of only gay activists. No more than 20% of the respondents belonged to a homosexual or an AIDS service organization. We also obtained responses from men who had sex with other men, although they did not identify as gay. Thus, we could make comparisons between different sub-populations represented in the sample.

Instruments. A primary concern underlying the GPS questionnaire is how AIDS has affected issues of lifestyle and sexuality. Besides the usual sociodemographic items (such as age, marital status, place of residence, occupation and education), questions were also included regarding to what degree subjects socialize with homosexual and heterosexual men. Other questions focused on sexual activity. Our primary goal in administering the GPS is gathering the necessary information so as to detect changes in sexual practices as a result of the AIDS epidemic and to construct a typology of risk-management strategies being employed by the respondents. The survey also attempts to gather additional information about risk-taking so as to establish correlations between lifestyle, social acceptance, sexual practices, relationships with partners, and the degree of protection adopted.

RESULTS AND DISCUSSION

Perceptions of social acceptance and diversity of lifestyles. The stigmatizing of gay people as a group was already an issue before the advent of AIDS. While repressive police measures with regard to homosexuality were already on the decline in the early eighties in France (Mossuz-Lavau, 1991), the appearance of AIDS led to the fear that gay men would be more strongly rejected by the general population, as they were being designated as a "group at risk" and therefore could be potentially blamed for a further spread of the epidemic. Quite fortunately this fear did not bear out in the reaction of the French; various polls and surveys (Moatti et al., 1995) point to the improved acceptance of homosexuality over the last several years. Since the initial 1985 GPS, an increasing number of respondents feel that their homosexuality is accepted by the people they know. And yet, despite a considerably more relaxed social environment over the past decade, some results from the Gay Press Survey temper undue optimism. Acceptance by family members is still a problem for a number of respondents: Only 25% of the men feel that their fathers accept them as a homosexual. Such acceptance is still rarer in the case of younger men (Schiltz, 1997), and open conflicts with family regarding love relationships are twice as severe among young gay men as among young people in the general population (Bozon & Villeneuve-Gokalp, 1995). This fear of conflict or rejection is compounded by the slow and sometimes difficult maturing process from the time one first realizes that he is attracted to men to the full acknowledgement of his sexual orientation.

The homosexual population is to be defined not only in terms of its minority status and particular sexuality, but also in terms of a specific lifestyle strongly influenced by sexual activity. About half of the respondents in the Gay Press Survey live in a relationship with another man, but it should be noted that one out of two homosexual couples live in an open relationship. The number of sexual partners among gay men is also much higher than that of the general population. According to data from the national survey on sexual behavior in France (ACSF), heterosexual men report having had 1.15 partners over the last twelve months, while respondents to the Gay Press Survey from the same age group report 14.1 partners. The ACSF documents as well a lower number of partners for bisexuals, with their reporting 2.8 partners of the same sex and 1.3 female partners (Messiah & Mouret-Fourme, 1995). Compared to the national random sample, the self-selected subjects of the GPS stand out, therefore, in terms of their number of sexual partners. This particular feature of the Gay Press Survey sample must be kept in mind so as not to confuse our subjects with homosexual men in general, given that our subjects tend to have a large number of sexual partners and tend to have lifestyles which are strongly influenced by their sexual orientation.

Over the years, our survey data have shown that the living situations of our gay male subjects vary a great deal (Pollak & Schiltz, 1990; Schiltz, 1993; Schiltz & Adam, 1995). In addition to their different social positions, homosexual men have highly diverse partnering and sexual lifestyles. Some men live alone, having few or many sexual partners; others live in an exclusive relationship, while still others have more casual encounters. Additional factors influence lifestyle, such as closeness to or distance from large gay communities and the level of tolerance found within the local social environment. It is, in fact, difficult to compare a homosexual man living in a small town fairly isolated from gay culture with a middle-class homosexual man whose life revolves around Paris' gay scene.

Having provided this brief review of the specificity and diversity of sociosexual lifestyles within our sample, we will now focus on how the subjects have adjusted to the risk for HIV infection.

Adjustment to HIV risk. In 1985, only 44% of the respondents stated that they were more cautious in their sexual behavior because of HIV (Pollak, Schiltz & Laurindo, 1986). This proportion surged to 80% by 1988 and has remained steady ever since (Schiltz, 1997). In addition, a consistent 11% of the gay men in the sample report always practicing safer sex (including men who have never had anal sex, before or since AIDS). So, it may be said that a total of nine men out of ten were engaging in safer practices in 1995.

Early in the epidemic, preventive practices were strongly associated with the degree of personal closeness to HIV-positive persons ($p < 0.001$), and an upper-level employment status ($p < 0.001$). Social gaps are gradually narrowing, however, except for men of a lower economical status, where the lower income was associated with higher rates of infection ($p < 0.001$; see also Bochow, 1997; Dowsett, Davis & Connel, 1992). Although initially exhibiting more higher risk behaviors, young people (less than 25 years old) have progressively adapted to risk since 1987, with their level of protection no longer differing from that of their elders, except for the youngest respondents (less than 20) who tend to not protect themselves at the time of their first sexual experiences.

The adjustment to risk found in our samples has consisted of using condoms during anal sex or eliminating anal penetration all together, as well as reducing the number of sexual partners and avoiding certain places for meeting men. We have observed that awareness of the extent of the epidemic among homosexual men has led to a significant reduction in partner-seeking (*cruising*) activity. Such cautiousness has an impact, of course, on the number of partners and the way couples choose to live. Whereas in 1985, 27% of the respondents reported over ten partners in six months, this rate fell to 16% in 1987 (Pollak & Schiltz, 1990). In 1985, 69% of the men living in a couple tolerated sexual partners outside the relationship, but only 48% of them did so in 1987 (i.e., a 21% drop over a two-year period).

In the early 1990s, advertising targeted at homosexual men, consisting exclusively of promoting the use of condoms, may have affected behavior. Between 1991 and 1995, a significant rise in sexual activity was counterbalanced by a significant increase in the proportion of respondents who regularly used condoms with their casual partners. Thus, in 1995, 34% of the respondents reported over ten partners in the course of the year compared with 31% in 1993 and 27% in 1991; 83% practiced penetration with their casual partners compared with 81% in 1993 and 71% in 1991;

and 73% protected themselves systematically in cases of anal penetration with casual partners compared with 64% in 1993 and 53% in 1991, that is, 20 points more over four years. This trend was confirmed by other indicators as well; over that same period, we have observed a sharp decrease in avoidance strategies which consist in limiting the number of partners or performing only certain sexual practices with casual partners. A revival of gay cruising has gone hand-in-hand with increasingly systematic protection as far as anal penetration is concerned. The limitation and selection of practices, places, and partners reached a high point in 1991. Since then, an increasing number of homosexual men have relied exclusively on safer sex practices. These overall indicators provide a measure of the impact of the preventive messages which promoted *condom use every time* starting in the 1990s. But the patterns reported thus far mask the complex risk avoidance strategies adopted by gay men during this period.

Differentiated adjustment to HIV risk: Sexual behavior and partner cofactors of condom use. Condom use varies widely depending on sexual practice and the kind of partner involved. Condom use is not the rule for fellatio; whereas, for anal penetration, condoms are often used. As far as fellatio is concerned, gays have resorted to a different kind of protection. In 1995, half of the respondents said they avoid letting any semen come into their mouths when they have sex with their steady partner. This risk avoidance practice has become even more common with casual partners, jumping from 52% of the sample in 1991 to 75% in 1995.

Protection in cases of penetration also increased significantly in relation to casual encounters (73% of the sample in 1995 as opposed to 53% in 1991); whereas, it remains fairly unchanged with steady partners (from 38% in 1991 to 44% in 1995).

These data show that, besides safer sex (adopting an array of protective practices and/or giving up risky practices all together),[1] French gay men have, in part, based their risk-reduction strategy on the stability of the relationship with their sexual partner. With casual partners, 89% of the respondents had given up anal intercourse or used a condom regularly. With stable partners, only 55% always used a condom or had given up anal intercourse. This difference in terms of protection can be attributed to *negotiated safety* (Kippax, Crawford, Davis, Roden & Dowsett, 1993) based on the fact that 87% of our French respondents had taken the AIDS antibody test and that their strategy for managing risk takes into account their own and their partners' HIV-status. Our observations also suggest that gays who live as a couple are more motivated to take the test. Depending on the test result, men decide how to behave in terms of HIV risk.

Most HIV-negative men who are in a steady relationship with a seronegative partner have given up protection strategies altogether: Over two-thirds of them used no protection at the time of their last anal penetration.

Keogh and Beardsell (1997) showed that HIV-positive gay men tend to disregard doctors' warnings as to the dangers of re-infection from HIV-positive sexual partners. Our observations confirm this tendency: one quarter of the HIV-positive couples from the Gay Press Survey say they use no precaution whatsoever. In contrast, safer sex is part of everyday life for most serodiscordant couples, especially when the uninfected partner has confirmed his status through an HIV test. Our observations about actual sexual practice show that, as with other groups (Giami & Schiltz, 1996), the decision to use a condom in couples is based on selective reasoning. Different sexual partners are treated differently by the same subject, and several other reasons come into play when partners who know each other are deciding to protect themselves or not. Respondents to our surveys increasingly tend to make distinctions based on the kind of bond they have with their sexual partners, and the way they handle risk in an intimate relationship depends greatly on their respective serological status.

These different kinds of protection based on the practice and partner involved also point out that condom use is only one element in risk management.

Differentiated adjustment to HIV risk: Coping strategies: Protection during intercourse and/or limiting risky situations. Another set of GPS questions enabled us to detect the diversity of behavioral strategies used to cope with the AIDS epidemic. While the items do not take into account all possible responses, the questions did enable us to detect four major risk-management strategies (of varying effectiveness, from an epidemiological point of view).

Some respondents try to reduce risk of exposure by changing their sexual lifestyle (e.g., reducing the number of partners, not having penetration with casual partners); others rely on preventive measures during intercourse (no penetration without condoms). These two kinds of risk management may be either isolated or combined. Thus, in the 1995 survey: (1) 27% of the respondents managed risk through preventive measures in sexual encounters only and did not try to limit situations of exposure; (2) 45% of the men combined the use of condoms with a change of lifestyle; (3) 11% of the respondents used no protection with their steady partners, 7% because they were monogamous, while others (4%) decided to use no protection as a couple, but to use condoms regularly with casual partners; (4) Despite prevention campaigns, a minority of the men (7%) opted for a strategy in which they selected their partners and places of encounter and used no other form of protection. Finally, a minority claimed not to have changed anything in their sexual lives, in spite of the risks incurred (5%), or claimed to have no strategy for avoiding risk (3%). These observations show that about 15% of the respondents either find it difficult to protect themselves efficiently or, for some other reason, still pursue risky behavior.

Continuing HIV risk behavior. Despite the effort to adapt to the epidemic, risky behavior still occurs. The percentage of individuals in the gay community who have adopted safer sex is high, but far from satisfactory. As demonstrated above, risky behavior still occurs among respondents. Since social communities tend to mediate risk, members consider the very fact of belonging to be a *protective envelope* (Douglas & Calvez, 1990). This holds for homosexual men, as well. However, some gay representatives from AIDS service organizations tend to think that a *residual risk* subsists mainly on the fringes of the gay scene; that is, among men not integrated into the community. We therefore tested if there was indeed more risk among these men.

In our sample, 9% of the respondents defined themselves as *heterosexual* or *bisexual*.[2] However, they did not report either more or fewer "risky penetrations" in the previous year than gays. Moreover, only 8% of the individuals in this group said they were HIV-positive, as opposed to 17% among self-identified gay men. This relatively lower prevalence of HIV cannot be attributed to a narrower sexual repertory. However, bisexual and heterosexual men do tend to have fewer sexual partners than self-identified gay men. Twenty-two percent of the bisexually- and heterosexually-identified men had more than ten partners during the previous year, compared with 35% of the homosexually-identified men. The bisexual and heterosexual men in the sample are also in sexual networks and geographical areas where HIV incidence is lower. In effect, most of these respondents lived outside the Paris region (63% vs. 55% for homosexual men), where the proportion of the HIV-positive men in the GPS is lower than in Paris (13% vs. 20%).[3] Therefore, it is too restrictive to single out *men less integrated in the gay community who have intercourse with other men without identifying as gay* as the absolute target for prevention campaigns. Even bisexuality among youth appears to be a *risk factor* only when it combines with other circumstances, such as coming from a lower social class, and perhaps being isolated or feeling less accepted because of one's homosexuality.

According to our observations, taking risks for HIV is not limited to the margins of the community. Well-informed men who practice safer sex also take risks. In 1995, as in previous surveys, one respondent out of five had engaged in unprotected anal intercourse in the last twelve months with a partner whose HIV-status was unknown or different from his own. Risky behavior is also not limited to the minority of men who never adapted effectively to the epidemic or men who gave up all protection systems after previously adopting safer sex (both groups combined making up only 2% of the sample). Even among the men who said they always engaged in safer sex or restricted sexual acts to mutual masturbation or petting, 17% reported at least one episode of risky behavior during the year.

Cruising associated with HIV risk. The number of homosexual men who stated that they had unprotected anal intercourse with partners of an unknown or different serological status is directly proportional to the number of partners, regardless of the respondent's risk-reduction strategies. Thus, 35% of the men who had more than 20 partners report having had unprotected anal penetration as opposed to 25% of those who had between 10 and 20 partners and 15% of those who had fewer than 10 partners in the last year. This trend suggests that a lifestyle centered on cruising multiplies the situations where one might experience problems with condoms themselves (such as a condom bursting) or other problems with safer sex, possibly due to psychological reasons.

Social science researchers, mainly American (Ekstrand, Stall, Kegeles, Hays, De Mayo & Coates, 1993; McCusker, Stoddard, McDonald, Zapka & Mayer, 1992; Stall, Ekstrand, Pollack, McKusick & Coates, 1990) and Dutch (de Wit & van Griensven, 1994), have observed breaches in the protection strategies of men who had previously closely followed safer sex precepts. To account for the occurrence of an episode of risky behavior among these men, these researchers coined the term *relapse* in order to describe men who had initially adopted safer practices, but who reverted back to unprotected sex. Previously, this term had been found most commonly in the American literature pertaining to substance use and treatment. In adopting the word *relapse*, unprotected sex was being implicitly compared to substance abuse, the underlying idea being that a single relapse sufficed for being *hooked* again on a chronic pathological behavior[4] (see Ekstrand, 1992; McCuster et al., 1992). Several European researchers studying HIV risk and sexuality have strongly criticized this approach[5] (Bochow, 1991; Davies & the Project SIGMA, 1992; Hart, Boulton, Fitzpatrick, McLean & Dawson, 1992).

The majority of European investigators have avoided associating sexuality with pathology, and have considered the *zero risk* objective of other HIV prevention programs to be unattainable, since a breach in one's system of protection could always occur due to many human reasons. It is not realistic to expect gay men, or others, to have 100% effective strategies which prevent every incident of risk-taking regarding HIV infection. This view, which we consider to be more realistic, leads us to recognize that all prevention systems constructed by individuals are imperfect, but that they are more effective than no prevention at all.

Our results show that the frequency of risky behavior depends on the stability of the relationship between partners. Generally with steady partners, when risky behavior exists, two-thirds of the risky acts occur regularly (at least once a month), except in the case of couples in which one of the partners has tested HIV-negative and the other HIV-positive, in which case two-thirds of the incidents reported occur only sporadically. When such a risk occurs with casual partners, the risk behavior appears to be more often due to a breach in the system of protection, that is, due to some imperfection in the prevention strategy: 80% of the respondents who took risks with casual partners did so less than four times a year. Therefore, for many who adopt safer sex, a 100% effective system of protection is very hard to maintain.

The above observations illustrate that for most of the men who adopted safer sex, risk-taking is often sporadic and in this sense may not be equated with the absence of all means of protection. Furthermore, in circumstances where partners trust each other, the abandoning of protected sex should not categorically be considered risky. Any examination of the frequency of risk-taking disproves the notion that prevention is no longer a major concern among gays. There is no support for the idea that French gay men have somehow *relapsed* into a state of no longer wanting to protect themselves.

CONCLUSION

Since 1985, our surveys show that differences still exist among French gay men in terms of behavior adjustments due to the epidemic, even though these differences have considerably lessened over time. Our results call into question the idea that the greatest risk for HIV is to be found in segments of the population which are less integrated in the gay community; well-informed men who have adopted safer sex also take risks.

The 1995 survey confirms the 1991 observation that safer sex practices stabilized at a high level, but this has not been enough to curb the epidemic among gays. As in earlier years, one respondent out of five reported unprotected anal penetration in the course of the year with a partner whose serological status was unknown or different from his own. Attributing this risk-taking to a relapse phenomenon would distort the reality of French gay men's sexuality. In point of fact, according to our observations, very few men have given up all means of protection after having practiced safer sex.

Results from this last survey also disprove the widely held belief that risk persists strictly on the margins of the *community*–particularly among men who have sex with other men but do not identify as gay–but also among the young and those who are socially disadvantaged. These sociodemographic factors appear to predispose to risk only when they are combined. Our results show that risk is more dispersed in the gay population than often thought, with self-identified gay men not being without risky behavior. In fact, even the behavior of many well-informed men who have opted for safer sex shows that it is not always easy to maintain a totally effective protection system. However, this does not mean that these men turn their back on prevention altogether.

Given the widespread risk of HIV-infection, prevention campaigns must target homosexual and bisexual men in all their diversity while reminding self-identified gay men that they should remain cautious. The aim is to keep promoting safer sex while recognizing its limits and taking into account the difficulty of maintaining such practices over a long period of time.

Whereas HIV prevention messages often urge people to protect themselves regardless of the situation and no matter who the sexual partner may be, it is a fact that over the past decade, respondents have been increasingly basing their protective practices on the level of emotional bonding with their sexual partner. They likewise take into account similar or dissimilar serological statuses. The analysis of how gay men react to risk as a couple shows that they want to know about their actual risk and to behave rationally in the face of the information. When in a chosen relationship, two partners who know that they are HIV-negative may decide not to protect themselves as a result of their commitment to each other or based on regular use of condoms with outside partners. This decision may be viewed as rational, and it may be concluded that most of those unprotected sexual practices cannot be deemed risky.

The prevention model targeted at the *gay community* encouraged gays to practice safer sexual behavior on all occasions. It was based on the notion that all men are equal when it comes to HIV risk, regardless of type of sex, who the partner is, or the circumstances of the sexual act. Yet despite the fact that the rule was often ignored, it should be recalled that fifteen years after the first AIDS cases were identified, a majority of respondents succeeded in avoiding sexually transmitted infections, including HIV.

A new analysis of the complex infection-avoiding strategies developed by gay men is needed. HIV/STD prevention should no longer be a matter of re-education aimed at helping everyone to adopt a single pattern of response to the epidemic. We need to attempt to adjust HIV/STD prevention messages, based on empirical data, to the whole range of lifestyles and norms. The goal is to approach risk management as it relates to an increasingly differentiated group of strategies chosen by gay men themselves on the basis of the bond which ties them to their partner and on the basis of their respective serological statuses. So far, no prevention advice in France has helped men in this decision-making process. At a time when combination therapies are changing the lives of HIV-positive homosexual men and, consequently, that of their partners, a more pragmatic approach could serve to develop more specific messages which would help gay men choose their own lifestyles and ways of managing risk, while still warning them of the specific difficulties implicit in those choices.

NOTES

1. French homosexual men definitely preferred the first option; only a minority gave up anal intercourse. In 1991, only 16% of homosexual men did not engage in anal intercourse with their steady partner, with 32% not having anal sex with a casual partner. Compared with other European countries, more homosexual men in France appear to prefer anal intercourse. For example, among Dutch homosexual men, a significant minority had given up anal intercourse (see Bochow et al., 1994). Michael Pollak (1991) explained these differences based on differences in prevention messages; whereas using condoms was recommended nearly everywhere in Europe, the major preventive strategy in the Netherlands called for abandoning anal intercourse.

2. The oft used term *bisexuality* covers a range of situations (Mendès-Leite, 1996). Some bisexuals lead a heterosexual lifestyle: they are married, live with a wife and may even have children. Others are single. Among the young, bisexual behaviour frequently occurs during the period of uncertainty before sexual preferences are stabilized.

3. The area where one lives is not the only explanatory factor, given that HIV contamination among bisexuals is always much lower: thus in comparable living areas, 14% of the bisexuals living in the Paris region are contaminated as opposed to 20% of the gays in Paris. These rates are respectively 5% and 11% in the provinces (that is, in regions outside of Paris).

4. Studies of addictive behaviour (such as nicotine poisoning, bulimia and alcoholism) have shown that sustaining changes is harder than making the initial decision to stop (McCusker, Stoddard, McDonald, Zapka & Mayer, 1992).

5. For more information about this point, see the AIDS Journal which provided ample coverage of the controversy (for example AIDS, 1992-1994, espe-

cially Davies, 1993; de Wit & van Griensven, 1994; de Wit, van Griensven, Kok & Sandfort, 1993; Ekstrand, 1992; Ekstrand, Stall, Kegeles, Hays, de Mayo & Coates, 1993; McCusker et al., 1992). There is also a useful discussion by Hart and Boulton (1995) regarding the theoretical stakes of this debate.

REFERENCES

Béjin, A. & Pollak, M. (1977). La rationalisation de la sexualité. *Cahiers Internationaux de Sociologie, LXII*:105-125.

Bell, A. P. & Weinberg, M. S. (1978). *Homosexualities. A Study of Diversity Among Men and Women.* New York: Simon and Schuster.

Bochow, M. (1991). Le safer sex: une discussion sans fin. Quelques remarques au sujet de la discussion actuelle. In M. Pollak, R. Mendès-Leite & J. van dem Borghe, eds., *Homosexualités et Sida*. Lille: Cahiers Gai-Kitsch-Camp.

Bochow, M. (1997, June). The prevalence of HIV among gay men as a function of socio-economic status. Oral presentation at the AIDS Impact Conference, Melbourne, Australia.

Bochow, M., Chiarotti, F., Davies, P., Dubois-Arber, F., Dür, W., Fouchard, J., Gruet, F., McManus, T., Markert, S., Sandfort, T., Sasse, H., Schiltz, M.-A., Tielman, R. & Wasserfallen, F. (1994). Sexual behavior of gay and bisexual men in eight European countries. *AIDS Care*, 6(5):533-549.

Bozon, M. & Villeneuve-Gokalp, C. (1995). Les enjeux des relations entre générations à la fin de l'adolescence. *Population*, 49(6):1527-1556.

Dannecker, M. & Reiche, R. (1974). *Der gewöhnliche Homosexuelle*. Frankfurt: Fischer.

Davies, P. (1993). Safer sex maintenance among gay men: Are we moving in the right direction? *AIDS*, 7:279-280.

Davies, P. M. & the Project SIGMA (1992). On relapse: Recidivism or rational response? In P. Aggleton, G. Hart, P. Davies, eds., *AIDS: Rights, Risk and Reason*. London: The Falmer Press, 133-140.

de Wit, J. B., van Griensven, J. P., Kok, G. & Sandfort, T. G. M. (1993). Why do homosexual men relapse into unsafe sex? Predictors of resumption of unprotected anogenital intercourse with casual partners. *AIDS*, 7:1113-1118.

de Wit, J. B. F. & van Griensven, J. P. (1994). Time from safer sex to unsafe sexual behavior among homosexual men. *AIDS*, 8:123-126.

Douglas, M. & Calvez, M. (1990). The self as a risk-taker. *Sociological Review*, 38(3): 951-962.

Dowsett, G. W., Davis, M. D. & Connel, R. W. (1992). Working class homosexuality and HIV/AIDS prevention: Some recent research from Sydney, Australia. *Psychology and Health*, 6:313-324.

Ekstrand, M., Stall, R., Kegeles, S., Hays, R., De Mayo, M. & Coates, T. (1993). Safer sex among gay men: What is the ultimate goal? *AIDS*, 7:281-282.

Ekstrand, M. L. (1992). Safer sex maintenance among gay men: Are we making any progress? *AIDS*, 6:875-877.

Gagnon, J. (1973). Male Homosexuality. In J. Gagnon & W. Simon, eds., *Sexual Conduct*. Chicago: Aldine.

Giami, A. & Schiltz, M.-A. (1996). Representation of sexuality and relations between partners: Sex research in France in the era of AIDS. *Annual Review of Sex Reseach*, 1-33.

Hart, G., Boulton, M., Fitzpatrick, R., McLean, J. & Dawson, J. (1992). Relapse to unsafe sexual behavior among gay men: A critique of recent behavioral HIV/AIDS research. *Sociology of Health and Illness*, *14*(2):216-232.

Hart, G. & Boulton, M. (1995). Sexual behavior in gay men: Towards a sociology of risk. In P. Aggleton, P. Davies, G. Hart, eds., *Safety, Sexuality and Risk*. London: Falmer Press, 55-67.

Keogh, P. & Bearsell, S. (1997). Sexual negotiation of HIV-Positive Gay Men. In P. Aggleton, P. Davies, & G. Hart, eds., *AIDS: Activism and Alliances*. London: Taylor & Francis, 226-237.

Kippax, S., Crawford, J., Davis, M., Roden, P. & Dowsett, G. (1993). Sustaining safe sex: A longitudinal study of a sample of homosexual men. *AIDS*, 7: 257-263.

Lot, F., Pillonel, J., Pinget, R., Cazein, F., Gouezel, P. & Laporte A. (1997). Diminution brutale du nombre de cas de sida. Rôle des nouvelles stratégies thérapeuthiques? *Bulletin épidémiologique hebdomadaire*, *11*:43-45.

McCusker, J., Stoddard, A. M., McDonald, M., Zapka, J. G. & Mayer, K. H. (1992). Maintenance of behavioral change in a cohort of homosexually active men. *AIDS*, 6:861-868.

Mendès-Leite, R. (1996). *Bisexualité. Le dernier tabou*. Paris: Calmann-Lévy.

Messiah, A., Mouret-Fourme, E. & the French National Survey on Sexual Behavior Group (1995). Sociodemographic characteristics and sexual behavior of bisexual men in France: Implications for HIV prevention. *American Journal of Public Health*, *85*(11):1543-1546.

Moatti, J. P., Grémy, I., Obadia, Y., Bajos, N., Doré, V. & Groupe KABP/ACSF (1995). SIDA: Dernière enquête nationale. *La Recherche*, *282*:30-34.

Mossuz-Lavau, J. (1991). Les lois de l'amour. Les politiques de la sexualité en France (1950-1990). Paris: Editions Payot.

Pollak, M. (1981). Les vertus de la banalité. *Le débat*, *10*:132-142.

Pollak, M. (1982). L'Homosexualité masculine ou le bonheur dans le ghetto? *Communications*, *35*:37-55.

Pollak, M. (1991). *AIDS Prevention for Men Having Sex with Men: Final Report to the European Community Concerted Action on Assessment of AIDS/HIV Preventive Strategies*. Lausanne: Institut de Médecine Sociale et Préventive (Cah. Rech. Doc IUMSP 75).

Pollak, M. & Schiltz, M.-A. (1987). Identité sociale et gestion d'un risque de santé. *Actes de la recherche en sciences sociales*, *68*:77-102.

Pollak, M. & Schiltz, M.-A. (1990). *Six années d'enquête sur les homo- et bisexuels masculins face au sida: 1985-1990*. Paris: Rapport à L'Agence Nationale de Recherche sur le Sida.

Pollak, M., Schiltz, M.-A. & Laurindo, L. (1986). Les homosexuels face à l'épidémie du SIDA. *Revue Epidémiologique et Santé Publique*, *34*:143-153.

Réseau National de Santé Publique (1997). La surveillance du sida en France. *Bulletin épidémiologique hebdomadaire*, *11*:46-49.

Schiltz, M.-A. (1993). *Les homosexuels masculins face au sida: Enquêtes 1991-1992*. Paris: Rapport à L'Agence Nationale de Recherche sur le Sida.

Schiltz, M.-A. (1997). Parcours homosexuels: Une sexualité non traditionnelle dans des réseaux d'échanges sexuels à forte prévalence du VIH. *Population*, *52*:6.

Schiltz, M.-A. & Adam, P. (1995). *Les homosexuels face au sida: Enquête 1993 sur les modes de vie et la gestion du risque VIH*. Paris: Rapport à L'Agence Nationale de Recherche sur le Sida.

Schiltz, M.-A. & Adam, P. (1996). Le test de dépistage au VIH: Diffusion parmi les homo- et bisexuels français. In *Le dépistage du VIH: Politiques et pratiques*. Paris: ANRS (Collection Sciences sociales et sida).

Spira, A., Bajos, N. & ACSF Group (1994). *Sexual Behavior and AIDS*. Aldershot, Avebury.

Stall, R., Ekstrand, M., Pollack, M., McKusick, L. & Coates, T. J. (1990). Relapse from safer sex: The next challenge for AIDS prevention efforts. *Journal of Acquired Immune Deficiency Syndromes [AIDS]*, *3*:1181-1187.

World Health Organization (1995). *AIDS-Surveillance in Europe*. Report No. 7.

The Importance of Contextualizing Research: An Analysis of Data from the German Gay Press Surveys

Michael Bochow, PhD

SUMMARY. A comparative analysis of the effects of various forms of sexual relationship on the frequency of risk behavior was conducted among gay men in Germany who participated in a survey via the gay press in 1996 (n = 3048). Of the West Germans, 22.1% of the men had at least one act of unprotected anal intercourse with a partner whose status was unknown (in the twelve months preceding the survey) as compared to 25.7% of the East Germans. Unprotected anal intercourse without knowing the partner's HIV status is considerably more frequent in steady relationships. Although risk behavior does occur in the context of casual sexual encounters, this form of risk contact remains sporadic (one to four times in the twelve months preceding the survey). Unprotected anal intercourse between partners with differing HIV status was found among 3.1% of the West Germans and 3.7% of the East Germans. Differences according to type of partnership are less pronounced for these men. The data from the 1996 survey provide no support for younger gay men being at greater risk for HIV infection through sexual contact. For the under-21 age group, the percentage of men without anal-genital sexual experience is particularly high and the percentage of men having had a higher number of sexual partners (more than 20 over the last

[Haworth co-indexing entry note]: "The Importance of Contextualizing Research: An Analysis of Data from the German Gay Press Surveys." Bochow, Michael. Co-published simultaneously in *Journal of Psychology & Human Sexuality* (The Haworth Press, Inc.) Vol. 10, No. 3/4, 1998, pp. 37-58; and: *New International Directions in HIV Prevention for Gay and Bisexual Men* (ed: Michael T. Wright, B. R. Simon Rosser, and Onno de Zwart) The Haworth Press, Inc., 1998, pp. 37-58; and: *New International Directions in HIV Prevention for Gay and Bisexual Men* (ed: Michael T. Wright, B. R. Simon Rosser, and Onno de Zwart) Harrington Park Press, an imprint of The Haworth Press, Inc., 1998, pp. 37-58. Single or multiple copies of this article are available for a fee from The Haworth Document Delivery Service [1-800-342-9678, 9:00 a.m. - 5:00 p.m. (EST). E-mail address: getinfo@haworthpressinc.com].

© 1998 by The Haworth Press, Inc. All rights reserved.

twelve months) is considerably less for men under-25 years than for the rest of the sample. *[Article copies available for a fee from The Haworth Document Delivery Service: 1-800-342-9678. E-mail address: getinfo@haworthpressinc.com]*

In the 1980s, the discussion about risk behavior led to the conclusion that not all gay men were equally affected by the disease. At the various international AIDS conferences and during European meetings, an increasing number of characteristics were identified which were purported to best define those most at risk (Bochow, 1990; Dannecker, 1990; Davies, Hickson, Weatherburn & Hunt, 1993; Kippax, Connell, Dowsett & Crawford, 1993; Pollak, 1988). Some of these risk factors included sexual inexperience and/or youth; poverty; alcohol and drug consumption; lack of acceptance of one's own homosexuality; and the specific affective and erotic nature of sexual interaction itself (Bochow, 1995). Using more colloquial language, the early research can be summarized thus: In addition to those who are very promiscuous, the gay men most at risk for HIV are those who are particularly timid, particularly poor, particularly drunk or high, particularly turned on by sex, and, last but not least, those men who are particularly uptight.

Which of these various *problem groups* has been the focus of prevention at any given time has been largely dependent on the interests and preferences of the particular social scientists or prevention activists involved. To a certain extent, it has also been a result of survey design, with different questionnaires focusing on different factors. Moatti, Beltzer, and Dab (1993) have discussed this topic in a well-thought-out article called *Models for the Analysis of HIV Risk Behavior: Approaches Restricted by Narrow Reasoning*, which includes a somewhat sarcastic commentary concerning the research and practice of HIV prevention. The authors question the value of particular statistical techniques, such as regression analysis, as they are used to determine the influence of specific independent variables on a dependent variable (in our case high-risk behavior). They argue that:

> The tendency to focus on one or another variable . . . can rather be traced to the specific competence or preference of the researcher, which is more related to the scholarly discipline of the scientist in question, than to an analysis of *reality* . . . Various publications stress the explanatory power of psychological aspects (personality structure), socio-psychological aspects (the meaning of the locus of control), . . . sociological aspects (the meaning of social support net-

works) . . . up to and including situation-specific aspects (differences of risks taken dependent on the specific parameters of sexual interaction) . . . A consequence of these approaches . . . is . . . that the mechanical limitations of the analyses are magnified, with the conclusions being rarely supported by critical reflection on the surrounding conditions of the behavior. The result is that elements of a different order are being investigated at one and the same level. These elements include biological variables [and] socio-demographic . . . or . . . psychological characteristics. The danger is great that, in the end, an exhaustive collection of hard data, coupled with an imposing statistical apparatus, produces highly tautological results, and that the presented pseudo-factors are nothing more than transformations of the dependent variables which they have set out to analyze and explain. In our opinion, the Anglo-American literature is full of such dead-end examples. (Moatti, Beltzer & Dab, 1993; pp. 1511-1512)

In a similar vein, Ludger Pientka, a German epidemiologist, has warned of inappropriate prevention policies based on analyses of risk factors:

The interventionist philosophy implicitly related to the risk factor approach causes great problems. There is a fundamental misunderstanding that groups to be targeted can be determined by means of statistical groupings defined by risk factors and social status. This *social fallacy* is caused by surmising that, by means of variables which have minor value for the social constitution of certain groups, causal and/or interventionist strategies can be developed. (Pientka, 1994; pp. 397-398)

The risk factor model (which is not exclusively of Anglo-American origin) has, as its goal, determining risk factors, that is, qualities of individuals or of specific groups which predispose them to having unprotected sex. These factors are then used to formulate interventions, messages and programs to promote stopping risk behavior through adopting protective practices and strategies, like condom use or abstinence. Such approaches labor under a double fallacy. First, that there is one, or at most a few, decisive factors *in the final analysis* which clarify and codify risk behavior. Secondly, that it is possible, having clarified and codified these factors, to influence the groups at risk so that they will never or only rarely indulge in risk behavior in the future.

Both of these fallacies, which seem remarkably resilient to criticism, are widespread–among scientists and others in AIDS prevention, alike.

Researchers are still dreaming of discovering a formula totally explaining risk behavior. The result is that the social sciences are forever rekindling the flames over the vexed question: Why do gay men (or persons in other social groups) in the nineties continue to become infected and what are the characteristics of these gay men (or heterosexual men or women)?

Fortunately, at the end of the Eighties a concept of risk minimization was proposed to counter the traditional model of risk elimination, the former concept having been adopted in an increasing number of countries, among them Australia, Germany and Great Britain (see Bochow, 1990; Dannecker, 1990; Davies et al., 1993; Kippax et al., 1993; Pollak, 1988). The prevention policy of minimizing, as opposed to eliminating, infection risks is based upon a realistic, but not fatalistic, understanding that human beings do not function like machines. We cannot be programmed or conditioned at will. In her keynote address at the Third International AIDS Impact Conference, Susan Kippax contrasted the *traditional* to the *socially informed* approach to prevention and prevention evaluation:

> Nowhere is the presence of interpretation more obvious than when we turn to the *outcome* variable, unsafe sexual practice. The difference between the traditional and social model rests, in the main, on whether unsafe sex is taken as any occurrence of unprotected anal intercourse or whether unprotected anal intercourse is contextualized in some way. (Kippax, 1997; p. 9)

The contexualization being referred to by Kippax will be demonstrated in the following analysis of data collected during the German Gay Press Survey conducted in 1996. This analysis will focus on the following three topics as they relate to risk-taking: type of partnership; risk-minimizing strategies; and younger age.

METHODS

Subjects. A total of 3,048 men participated (514 or 17% from East Germany, including East Berlin and 2,534 or 83% from West Germany, including West Berlin). Forty-five percent of the participants live in the four German cities with a population of one million or more (Berlin, Hamburg, Munich, and Cologne). Twenty-one percent of the participants live in cities and towns with less than 100,000 residents. The mean age of the participants is 34.9 years (median: 33). The highest level of education is distributed as follows (percentages represent the associated diploma or its equivalent): 11% primary school diploma, 24% 10th grade diploma, 65% pre-university diploma (39% have a university degree, 17% are college students). These percentages indicate that men having ended their education at primary school and those living in smaller cities and towns are underrepresented in the sample; however, there are enough participants from both of these groups to be included in the statistical analysis.

Instruments. In July 1996, for the fifth time since 1987, a four-page questionnaire was circulated by the most important gay magazines in Germany. The survey asked gay men about their sexual behavior under the impact of AIDS. This was a replication of the version of the survey that had been carried out in November 1991 and December 1993. All surveys were commissioned by the Federal Center for Health Education (Bundeszentrale für gesundheitliche Aufklärung) in Cologne.

It is still not possible to conduct a representative study of men who have sex with men, even for those men who identify as gay. In spite of substantial progress in Western and Central European societies, homosexual behavior continues to be a largely hidden phenomenon, with gay men being the focus of discrimination and marginalization (Bochow, 1997).

Given this limitation, measuring the behaviors and attitudes of gay German men in light of HIV has been particularly problematic. A nationwide survey conducted through the gay press has proven to be the best solution for obtaining valid and reliable data. Replication of the study at regular intervals since 1987, along with making use of interregional and international comparison of results, has ensured the quality of the data and a balanced interpretation of the findings.

The surveys conducted in 1987 and 1988 in West Germany along with those conducted in 1991, 1993, and 1996 in united Germany show a large degree of stability in the sociodemographic structure of the sample. The samples do, however, underrepresent gay men over 44 years old and men with little contact to the gay community (not only men in rural areas but also men in the cities who have little contact to community structures). The tendencies found in the surveys can, nevertheless, serve as indicators for trends over time among homosexually active men in Germany, as the men who are most active socially and sexually (the men who could be considered "trendsetters") are over-represented. As in France (Schiltz, 1993; Schiltz & Adam, 1995), the questionnaires were distributed through the gay press, as this is the most efficient method to obtain a large sample from all regions in the country. Interestingly, the results obtained reflect those found using the method of conducting standardized interviews as reported in Australia (Kippax et al., 1993) and the United Kingdom (Davies et al., 1993).

RESULTS

Type of Partnership

Type of Partnership and Anal Intercourse. All national studies of gay men in Germany since 1971 show that about four-fifths of the respondents practice anal intercourse at least *sometimes*, whether as the receptive partner, as the insertive partner, or playing both roles (see Bochow, 1988, 1994; Dannecker, 1990; Dannecker & Reiche, 1974). In 1996, 81% of the West Germans surveyed and 82% of the East Germans had at least occasional anal-genital contact. The percentage of men who did not practice anal intercourse in the last twelve months is highly dependent on the relationship status of the subjects. Twenty-seven percent of the men without a steady partner at the time of the study reported no anal-genital contact; whereas, only 15% of the men in a closed (monogamous) relationship and 10% of the men in open (non-monogamous) relationships did not have anal intercourse over the last year.

Fifty-four percent of the men practiced both receptive and insertive anal intercourse. Ten percent had exclusively receptive and 17% exclusively insertive anal sex. The flexibility of the sexual repertoire is also dependent on the partnership status of the subjects. Forty-five percent of the men who were not in a steady relationship had both receptive and insertive contact; whereas, 58% of the subjects in (for the most part) monogamous partnerships and 65% of those in non-monogamous relationships played both roles during anal intercourse. The proportion of men who have exclusively insertive or receptive sex is not dependent on relationship status.

Not only the incidence of sexual contact, but also its frequency, appears to be dependent on type of relationship. In looking at all sexual practices as a whole, we find that 42% of the men in steady partnerships had sexual contact several times a week; whereas, only 14% of the men not in a primary relationship had sex this often. Thirty-five percent of the men in steady partnerships had sex several times a month with their primary partner or with other partners; only 24% of the men without a steady partner had sexual contact with this frequency. This indicates that three fourths (77%) of the men in primary relationships had sex several times a month or more often, whereas only 38% of the men without steady partners reported this frequency of sexual contact.

In analyzing anal-genital contacts there appear to be even greater differences based on partner status. Thirty-seven percent of the men in steady relationships (representing 20% of the total sample) had anal-genital contact several times a month or several times a week. Fifteen percent of the men not in a steady relationship (representing 12% of the total sample) had anal-genital contact with this frequency. When all responses are tabulated we find that 27% of the sample had frequent anal-genital contact. (The figures 20% and 12% cannot simply be added because 5% of all respondents had frequent anal sex with both their steady partner and other partners). This percentage is comparable to that found in the wave of the national survey administered in 1993 (Bochow, 1994).

Frequency of Risk Behavior and Type of Partnership. Only 21 men (0.7% of the sample) did not respond to the question regarding unprotected anal intercourse with partners whose HIV status they did not know, and 38 men (1.2% of the sample) did not answer the follow-up question regarding which partner was involved and at what frequency the unprotected sex occurred.

Seventy-seven percent of the West Germans and 74% of the East Germans reported not having had unprotected anal intercourse in the last twelve months with a partner whose HIV status they did not know. Ninety-six percent of both the West and East German samples did not have unprotected anal intercourse with a partner whose HIV status was different than their own. A total of 76.4% of the West Germans and 72.4% of the East Germans did not have either of these two forms of risk contact in the last year. As compared to 1993, this represents a stable pattern of safer sex behavior among the West Germans (no risk contacts in 1993: 75.9%) and a slight increase in safer sex behavior among the East Germans (no risk contacts in 1993: 70.3%). When looking at safer sex compliance trends since 1987, the picture shown in Table 1 emerges.

The results of the studies conducted in 1991 and 1993, as well as the results of other research in Germany (Dannecker, 1990) and in Western Europe (Bochow et al., 1994; Davies et al., 1993; Schiltz, 1993; Schiltz & Adam, 1995), show that anal intercourse, including unprotected anal intercourse, occurs predominantly in steady partnerships (Bochow, 1994). Re-

TABLE 1. Subjects with No Risk Contacts

Year of Survey	West Germans %	East Germans %
1987	61	(no data available)
1988	63	(no data available)
1991	69	59
1993	76	70
1996	76	72

garding the structure and meaning of anal sex among gay men see the pertinent analysis of de Zwart, van Kerkof and Sandfort (1995).

The results of the German survey in 1996 strongly support the above observation. Twelve percent of all subjects report unprotected anal-genital contact with a steady partner whose HIV status was unknown to them. This risk was taken by 5.5% of the total sample once a month or more often as shown in Table 2. Nine percent of the men surveyed had unprotected anal intercourse with non-steady partners whose status was unknown to them (excluding anonymous encounters). This risk was taken by 0.7% of the men (20 subjects) once a month or more often. Eleven percent of the men had anonymous unprotected anal sex with partners of unknown status. This situation was reported by 0.6% of the sample (20 subjects) as having occurred once a month or more often.

These data show that a significant percentage of the men (23%) have risk contacts with partners whose serostatus is unknown to them. The percentages also clearly indicate that, for the large majority of men who risk HIV infection (four-fifths), taking risk with non-steady partners is a sporadic occurrence (one to four times a year). This observation makes clear how meaningless it is to describe such sporadic events as *relapse into unsafe behavior*. For the men who report one to four unsafe sexual contacts with casual or anonymous partners, most of their sexual behavior actually consists of protected anal intercourse, mutual masturbation, or oral sex. The sporadic risk contacts are, therefore, exceptions which do not represent a *relapse* or return into a phase of increased unprotected behavior.

Even in steady partnerships, risk-taking in terms of HIV infection is rather the exception than the rule. The highest frequency of risk contacts is, however, found among this group. Of the men in steady partnerships who engaged in risk-taking: 46% had risk contacts once a month or more often, 16% five to ten times, and only 38% had sporadic risk contacts (i.e., one to four times in the last twelve months).

As noted above, 23% of the respondents (26% of the East Germans and 22% of the West Germans) had at least one incident of unprotected anal-genital contact with a partner of unknown serostatus. A much smaller percentage of men (3.2%) reported unprotected anal intercourse with partners whose serostatus was different from their own (3.5% of the East Germans, 3.1% of the West Germans). These highest risk contacts also take place at a higher frequency within the context of the steady relationship. However, the differences related to partner status are not as great for serodiscordant encounters as for sex with partners of unknown status.

Condom Use As a Regular Part of Sexual Practice. Four-fifths of the men (78%) who had anal sex in the last year with non-steady partners

TABLE 2. Anal Intercourse Without a Condom, Serostatus of Sex Partner Unknown (in the 12 months preceding the survey; 1996)

	N	%
Yes	693	22.7
No	2,334	76.6
No Response	21	0.7
Total	3,048	100.0
With steady partner		
1-4 times	141	4.6
5-10 times	57	1.9
Every month/week	168	5.5
Not applicable	2,682	87.9
Total	3,048	100.0
With casual partners		
1-4 times	217	7.1
5-10 times	42	1.4
Every month/week	20	0.7
Not applicable	2,731	90.8
Total	3,048	100.0
With anonymous partners		
1-4 times	282	9.2
5-10 times	26	0.9
Every month/week	19	0.6
Not applicable	2,721	89.2
Total	3,048	100.0

reported that they always use condoms during anal intercourse. It can be stated that these men have integrated condom use as a regular part of their sexual practice. A further 15% of these men reported that they use condoms frequently. These respondents can be described as having adopted condom use as part of their sexual practice, but condom use each time is not a given. Eighty-five percent of the men in the sample reported using a condom during their last act of anal intercourse with a non-steady partner. There are no differences regarding frequency of condom use based on role played during intercourse (receptive, insertive, or both).

Within steady partnerships there is a considerably smaller portion of men who regularly use condoms. Only one-third (35%) of the men who had anal sex with their steady partner always use a condom. Forty-six percent report never using condoms. Whether or not a condom is regularly used is dependent on the length of the steady relationship. Fifty-four percent of the men with relationships of one to six months always use a condom when having anal intercourse (29% never). Where the relationship has lasted seven to twelve months, the percentage of men regularly using condoms falls to 44%, with the percentage of men never using condoms rising to 38%. In relationships of over two years, regular condom use drops to one-fourth, and those never using condoms is at 56%. There is a similar trend concerning the use of condoms during the most recent act of anal intercourse with a steady partner.

Number of Partners and Risk Behavior. The relationship between a higher number of partners and the likelihood of risk contact, as first reported in 1993-1994, continues to find support in the data. Over four-fifths (84%) of the men with one to five sex partners in the last year had no risk contacts (unprotected anal intercourse with a partner of unknown or discordant serostatus). For men with six to fifty partners, this percentage falls to 72%. For men with over fifty partners, the figure is 61%. As shown in Table 3, men with a lower number of partners tend to have risk contacts with a steady partner, whereas, men with a higher number of partners have risk contacts with non-steady partners. For men with more than fifty partners there is a particularly high percentage of those who have risked HIV infection with both steady and non-steady partners.

In Table 4, the men are grouped according to frequency of risk contacts with partners with unknown serostatus, regardless of type of partnership. This was possible because information concerning the frequency of the risk contacts for all types of partners (steady, non-steady, and anonymous) was collected using the same method.

One to two risk contacts received the value 1.5; three to four risk contacts = 3.5; five to ten risk contacts = 7.5; risk contact every month = 14; risk contact every week = 60. It is likely that this method of calculation results in an underestimation of the total risk contacts for men with a high frequency of contacts. This potential problem is, however, not important for the purposes of this study; namely, the comparison of the individual subgroups: (1) men without risk contacts; (2) men with few/sporadic risk

TABLE 3. Number of Partners and Risk Contacts* in Preceding 12 Months

	Number of partners				
Risk Contacts	1-5	6-50	>50	Total	(No response)
	%	%	%	%	
No risk contacts	84	72	61	76	(n = 2213)
Risk contacts with casual partners only	4	15	24	11	(n = 311)
Risk contacts with steady partner only	10	6	5	8	(n = 222)
Risk contact with casual and steady partners	3	7	10	6	(n = 162)
Total N	1282	1364	262	2908	
Total %	44	47	9	100	

* Unprotected anal intercourse with partners of unknown or discordant serostatus

TABLE 4. Number of Partners and Frequency of Risk Contacts*

		Number of risk contacts						
Number of Partners	n	none	1-5	6-15	16-35	60-180	No	Total
		%	%	%	%	%	%	%
No partner	76	100	–	–	–	–	–	2.5
1 partner	477	85	5	5	–	4	2	15.6
2-5 partners	826	81	9	4	1	4	2	27.1
6-10 partners	478	75	15	6	2	2	1	15.7
11-20 partners	443	70	15	6	2	4	2	14.5
21-50 partners	459	72	16	5	1	5	1	15.1
51 or more partners	262	62	22	9	2	5	–	8.6
no response	27	85	11	4	–	–	–	0.9
Total N	3046	2332	370	158	36	114	38	
Total %		77	12	5	1	4	1	100.0

* Unprotected anal intercourse with partners of unknown or discordant serostatus

contacts; (3) men with frequent risk contacts; and (4) men with very frequent risk contacts.

Table 4 provides further support for the relationship between number of partners and the occurrence of risk contacts depicted in Table 3. Eighty-one percent of the men with two to five sex partners had no unprotected anal-genital contact with a partner of unknown serostatus. Only 62% of the men who had over fifty partners reported no risk contact of this kind. The main difference between the men with very few partners (2-5) and those with the highest number of partners (over 50) is the percentage of men with sporadic risk contacts (one to five times in the last twelve months). The majority of men with a high frequency of risk contacts had these contacts with their steady partner. This explains how the high frequency of risk contacts is relatively independent from the number of total partners.

The findings presented to this point concerning partnership and risk lead to the following conclusions: It is not the often discussed promiscuity of gay men in the 1980s–that is, their *fast lane* lifestyle of having multiple partners–which results in a high incidence of risk, but rather the psychosexual dynamic of the steady partnerships in which they are a part. The incidence of risk within steady partnerships is considerably higher than that within casual encounters. The affective dynamic of more intimate and committed sexual relationships excludes the distant, calculated risk management which can take place during casual sex.

The different dynamic of such intimate relationships, as opposed to more casual contacts, has been discussed in Germany (Dannecker, 1994) and in Sweden (Henriksson, 1995) using the term *risk factor love*, based on qualitative research which they conducted. Particularly, Dannecker has emphasized that permanent relationships often are accompanied by the fantasy of unity and permanence, regardless of whether the relationship proves to be a lasting one in reality. The feeling of love which develops, or which is at least fantasized, in steady relationships can nullify the more careful management of risk which one finds during casual sex. For gay men with permanent relationships, the condom may symbolize not only the presence of AIDS; it can also be seen as an unbearable barrier to intimacy with the partner. Both aspects can lead the partners to refrain from using the condom. Seen in this light, the desire for trust and intimacy, like the desire to escape the dictates of the prevention *commandments*, plays a much greater role in sexual interactions with steady relationships. The feeling of being kept apart by the condom is much easier to bear in sexual interactions outside of permanent relationships than in love relationships. The feeling of being in love temporarily neutralizes the impulses that exercise control. Therefore, the strong affective coloring of sexual interaction in a love relationship often leads to patterns of behavior that are different from those seen in casual sex. Casual sex interactions are much more open to conscious control and individual risk management. Of course, this does not mean that casual sex contacts are completely unproblematic as far as risk-taking behavior is concerned. Rewarding casual sexual interactions may contain the *promesse de bonheur* of a steady relationship. Permanent relationships and casual contacts are not separated by some insurmountable barrier. Fantasy is invariably a factor which can influence action. Even a fantasized intimacy can lead to risk-taking behavior during a casual sexual contact. The sexual fantasies that develop out of psychological and physical needs have to be taken into consideration in the analysis of sexual interactions, as does the influence of subconscious processes that are beyond conscious controls. Consequently, even in the case of casual sex, unprotected anal-genital contacts can mean that the distancing from the partner, which may be symbolized by the use of a condom, is being avoided (Bochow, 1995).

The campaign of ACON (AIDS Council of New South Wales, 1996) in Sydney for gay men who want to consider not using condoms in their relationship ("Talk, Test, Test again, Trust") represents a practical application of similar findings in Australia regarding partnership and risk (see Kippax, 1997). In future prevention campaigns for gay men in Germany (and perhaps in other countries, as well), the need for intimacy, trust, and togetherness–which are most deeply expressed in love relationships–need to be taken into account. Deficits concerning the management of risk in steady relationships need to be discussed. By focusing on the problems of risk management in couples, rather than the need for intimacy and connectedness, we avoid the danger of developing campaigns which de facto emphasize the importance of monogamy and faithfulness rather than addressing the dynamic risk itself.

Risk-Minimizing Strategies

When reviewing the common risk management strategies used to avoid HIV infection, three basic response patterns can be distinguished:

1. Selective Strategies. These consist of responses such as reducing the number of partners, avoiding certain pick-up locations or paying particular attention to the appearance of the prospective partner. Such selective strategies raise more problems than they solve; the protection they afford against HIV infection is purely illusory.

2. The Steady Relationship Strategy. This involves embarking either on a monogamous relationship or a relationship whose rule is only *safe sex* with partners other than the steady partner.
3. The Safer Sex Strategy. The last behavior pattern is the only one which merits being called a genuine *prevention strategy*. It is practiced by those who have *safer sex*, who have sexual contact exclusively with men of similar test status, or who limit their sexual activity to mutual masturbation.

The above strategies were identified based on the data from the national studies conducted through the gay press in France (Pollak & Schiltz, 1991; Schiltz & Adam, 1995) and in Germany (Bochow, 1994). In 1993, 72% of West Germans and 63% of East Germans reported that they either regularly apply the safer sex rules, have sex only with partners who have the same HIV status, or that they restrict their sex to the practice of mutual masturbation. Twelve percent of the West Germans and 17% of the East Germans believe that their steady partnership sufficiently protects them from an HIV infection. Six percent of the West Germans and 10% of the East Germans use a *selective* protection strategy in the belief that reducing the number of sexual partners and choosing partners carefully sufficiently reduces their risk (Bochow, 1994). The differences between West and East Germans, first observed in 1993, have lessened over time. In 1996, 6% of all respondents used a selective strategy; 8% placed trust in their steady partnership as the way to avoid infection; and 80% practiced safer sex on a more or less regular basis. Four percent of the respondents report that they have difficulties with safer sex or that they have no risk management strategy. (As a comparison, in the French survey of 1993, 73% of the respondents reported using safer sex as a way to reduce risk (protective strategy); 14% rely on their steady partnership; and 8% use a selective strategy (Schiltz & Adam, 1995).)

Which risk reduction strategy is employed depends on the relationship status of the respondent. Men in monogamous partnerships have an above-average tendency to use the partner selection strategy and the strategy of being in a steady relationship as ways to minimize their risk for HIV infection. Men in non-monogamous partnerships and those not in a steady relationship tend to use safer sex strategies. Almost two thirds of the men who either do not make use of a risk reduction strategy or who report difficulties keeping to safer sex rules are not in a steady partnership.

HIV-Testing and Risk-Minimizing Strategies. One of the questions in the 1996 survey focused on the motivation to have oneself tested for HIV. The possible responses included, *I would like to stop using a condom when having sex with my steady partner.* Twenty-seven percent of all respondents had themselves tested for HIV to find out if they had the same serostatus as their partner so they could stop using condoms in their relationship. But for men in steady relationships, this percentage is even higher, namely 38 percent. This high percentage is evidence of the large number of men who experience condom use as being a disruptive factor in the intimate relationship with their steady partner. In fact, not only men in steady partnerships report that condoms disrupt their sexual relations. Questions were included in the survey regarding attitudes toward condom use. For the sample as a whole, only one third of the men (34%) who had anal sex feel that condoms *do not disrupt* or *hardly disrupt* their sexual relations; whereas, one fifth (19%) feel very restricted and almost one half (46%) report a moderate level of disruption.

The Risk Behavior of Younger Gay Men

Since the late 1980s, the particular risk for HIV infection among younger gay men has been a topic of debate in both the United States and in Europe. The data from the 1996 survey in Germany reveal the following: Of the subjects under 21 years old there were only 65% who reported no risk contacts for the previous twelve months. This is compared to 77% of subjects aged 21-24, 75% of the men 25-29, and 76% of those 30-54 years of age. For those in the age group 21-29 there is, therefore, no evidence in the data for higher risk compared to those in the age group 30-54.

In analyzing the frequency of the risk contacts, we find that the youngest age group (16-20 year olds) actually had the least number of sexual encounters placing them at risk for HIV infection. For the under-21 age group, the percentage of men without anal-genital sexual experience is particularly high. The percentage of men having had a higher number of sexual partners (more than 20 over the last twelve months) is also considerably less for men under 24 than for the rest of the sample. All of these observations fail to provide support for younger gay men (including the group under 30 and, in a separate analysis, the group under 21) being at greater risk for HIV infection through sexual contact.

The Relationship Between Age and HIV Infection Rate. The data collected in the French national surveys since 1985 (Schiltz & Adam, 1995) and in the German surveys since 1987 indicate a constant trend of higher infection rates among older age groups. As this trend has not changed over time, this would seem to indicate that infection is a function of the length of a man's sexual career.

In the 1993 wave of the German Gay Press Survey, none of the West German (including West Berlin) subjects aged 16-20 who had been tested were infected. Whereas, 6.2% of subjects aged 21-24, 6.5% of men aged

25-29, and 10.8% of men aged 30-34 were HIV-positive. In the older age categories, the rate of infection was 15.1% for the 35-44 year olds and 18% for the men 45-54. A similar pattern could be observed in the 1991 data for Western Germany. Data from France for the period 1985-1993 also shows a stabile pattern of higher infection for the older age groups (Schiltz & Adam, 1995). What the trends in the data in both countries seem to indicate is that for the age cohorts which became adults during the epidemic, the likelihood of infection is a function of becoming older.

In 1993, 69% of the West German respondents had been tested; in 1996, this rose to 73%. For the men over 24 years old, the rate of being tested is slightly above these percentages; for those under 25, it is slightly lower. One explanation for the rise in infection rate with age could be that younger positive men do not take the test until they show symptoms of infection. Another interpretation would be that the self-selective nature of a written questionnaire distributed through the gay press is unlikely to reach those younger men who are least integrated into the community (and perhaps, therefore, at greater risk for infection). The latter explanation may be the case, for example, for a small, marginalized group of young, working-class men, who have left home, some of whom survive through prostitution. In Germany, however, this subpopulation is not large in number (Jürgen Meggers, Department of Health in Charlottenburg, Berlin; personal communication). Up to this point there is also no evidence that young Turkish, Kurdish, and Arab men are disproportionately infected (in contrast to young African-American and Latino men in the United States). There is a degree of ethnic segregation in Germany, but it has not had the same epidemiological consequences as segregation in the United States. As for the first interpretation suggested above concerning marginalized, working-class men, there is a lack of empirical data.

It is important to note that men who are particularly socially and sexually active in gay networks are over-represented in the gay press samples. This would indicate an over-representation of men who are HIV positive. In Germany, with a population of 82 million, an estimated 60,000-90,000 are infected. Further, the Robert Koch Institute estimates that two-thirds of infections (40,000 to 60,000 men total) are to be found among gay and bisexual men (AIDS/HIV, 1997). An estimated 1.2-1.4 million men in the country have same-sex relations. Therefore, it is clear that the infection rate is well under the 10-12% found in the survey samples. The effects of selection in the surveys tend to exaggerate the actual epidemiological situation among the gay population. Nevertheless, it is of relevance that the infection rate in the samples has risen for men over 20 years old in the period, 1993-1996. This trend most definitely exists, albeit not to the degree suggested by the data.

In the data from the 1996 wave of the German survey we see the first signs of infections leveling off in the men 30 and older. In that year there are also no infections reported by West Germans in the 16-20 year age group. Of the 21-24 year olds, 3.2% were infected, and of the men age 25-29, 7.7% were HIV-positive. The percentage of infected subjects age 30-34 rose to 12.2%, with the percentage of infected 35-44 year olds remaining constant (12.4%), and a slight increase for the 45-54 year old group (13.7%) being observed. In light of these trends, the constant rate of infection for the age group 30-54 can be counted as a success for AIDS prevention efforts, being a result of protective measures undertaken by the men of this group. Disturbing, however, is that 12% of the men become infected between the ages of 16 and 35 (given the consistent finding of no infection before age twenty and a prevalence of about 12% for the age group 30-34 (see Table 5)). This trend is believed to reflect the real pattern of new infections by age over time, in spite of the fact that the survey samples over-represent HIV-positive men.

CONCLUSION

Although steady partnerships theoretically provide the best relational context in which to negotiate safer sex, we find that higher risk behavior is more likely to occur in this type of relationship than in situations with anonymous partners. In terms of prevention programs for gay men, this means that the *negotiated safety* approach (see Kippax, 1997), which is also promoted in Germany, is in need of further development.

The Australian (and British) concept of negotiated safety recognizes the need which many gay men have to refrain from using condoms in their steady partnerships. Clarifying the HIV status of both partners is promoted as being the pre-requisite for not using a condom. Untested men are therefore encouraged to give up the practice of trying to guess the serostatus of steady partners, and to instead rely on testing as the first step when deciding to stop condom use. Testing alone, however, is not sufficient. The decision to stop using condoms must be part of a larger communication process which includes talking about sex outside of the relationship. Negotiated safety also promotes the use of condoms every time when having anal sex outside the partnership and/or the restriction of casual sex to lower risk behavior. The slogan for the negotiated safety campaign in Sydney is therefore "Talk, Test, Test again, Trust" (ACON Leaflet, 1996). It must be emphasized that negotiated safety does not address the problem of serodis-

TABLE 5. Serostatus of Tested West German Subjects by Age

Age	Year	HIV Negative n (%)	HIV positive n (%)	HIV no response n (%)	Total N (%)
16-20	1993	28 (93.3)	0 (0.0)	2 (6.7)	30 (100.0)
	1996	20 (100)	0 (0.0)	0 (0.0)	20 (100.0)
21-24	1993	165 (85.1)	12 (6.2)	17 (8.8)	194 (100.0)
	1996	116 (93.5)	4 (3.2)	4 (3.2)	124 (100.0)
25-29	1993	443 (85.0)	34 (6.5)	44 (8.4)	521 (100.0)
	1996	387 (90.0)	33 (7.7)	10 (2.3)	430 (100.0)
30-34	1993	333 (81.6)	44 (10.8)	31 (7.6)	408 (100.0)
	1996	393 (82.9)	58 (12.2)	23 (4.9)	474 (100.0)
35-44	1993	262 (79.2)	50 (15.1)	19 (5.7)	331 (100.0)
	1996	430 (82.2)	65 (12.4)	28 (5.4)	523 (100.0)
45-54	1993	113 (78.5)	26 (18.1)	5 (3.5)	144 (100.0)
	1996	159 (83.7)	26 (13.7)	5 (2.6)	190 (100.0)
55 +	1993	31 (79.5)	6 (15.4)	2 (5.1)	39 (100.0)
	1996	70 (85.4)	12 (14.6)	0 (0.0)	82 (100.0)
No Age Given	1993	5 (83.3)	1 (16.7)	0 (0.0)	6 (100.0)
	1996	2 (50.0)	1 (25.0)	1 (25.0)	4 (100.0)
Total	1993	1380 (82.5)	173 (10.3)	120 (7.2)	1673 (100.0)
	1996	1577 (85.4)	199 (10.8)	71 (3.9)	1847 (100.0)

cordant couples. The model does, however, seek to make the serodiscordance issue clear by promoting the process of communication and testing.

The structural problem with every form of HIV prevention as well as with every form of individual risk management strategy is the inherent contradiction between the desire for intimacy–which manifests itself in a need for love and its sexual expression–and the necessity to take distance, which is the prerequisite for successful risk management practices. There is no golden rule regarding how to deal effectively with these competing needs, any more than there are eternal truths to be learned in studying the psychosocial factors related to HIV-infection. In any event, the orthodox United States AIDS-prevention strategy promoted at international AIDS conferences leads up a blind alley. Insisting on condom use under all circumstances silences those men who do not see themselves able to heed the message of safer sex all the time. This in turn leads to risk-taking becoming a taboo subject, much as the topic of homosexual contacts was previously taboo. The global recommendation that all gay men should behave sexually as if they were positive creates more problems than it claims to solve. The message to use a condom *always, under all circumstances, and with every partner* when having anal intercourse is patronizing and infantilizing. Such a message denies gay men the opportunity to develop their own risk-avoidance and risk-reduction strategies–personalized approaches which reflect the details of their individual lives.

A behaviorist conditioning approach to HIV prevention which focuses on condom use compliance thus limits our understanding of real risk behavior and prevents the further development of concepts for prevention. HIV prevention models in current use can only be further refined if the dimensions of sexual communication and verbal communication are integrated. This does not mean just communication which is narrowly focused on HIV status, but also communication about failed attempts on the part of the couple to ensure the degree of safety they would like. Risk-taking takes place in a vast array of situations. In addition to taking place with particular (special) partners, many risk contacts arise from unique and highly specific sexual interactions which have a dynamic of their own. These interactions are often not amenable to a calculated risk management strategy. In order to explore in more detail the contexts of risk-taking, qualitative methods are necessary so as to go beyond the limits of quantitative models. This would allow a further contextualization of the risk reduction strategies employed by gay men. This article is an attempt at doing this type of contextualization.

Prevention also needs to integrate into the discourse a discussion of failed attempts at protecting oneself from HIV. Such a discussion would help gay men to avoid developing feelings of guilt and shame while promoting a process of communication about the problems men have with safer sex. Discussing how prevention strategies have not worked would also promote a contextualizing of risk-taking. A similar discussion among researchers would be equally fruitful so as to better understand the phenomena associated with HIV risk.

Contextualization can prove useful as well when analyzing the risk-taking of young gay men. For example, an analysis of the German survey from 1996 indicates that more of the 16-20 year olds risked infection than the rest of the sample. However, further examination of the data reveal that the youngest group of men had the lowest frequency of risk contacts, the lowest number of sex partners, and the highest number of men without anal sex experience. Such observations should not, of course, be construed as being true for all youth, given that young people are a very diverse group. In order to take into account the diversity of experience found among young men, highly differentiated research methods need to be employed which go beyond distribution of a survey like the one presented here. Only by gathering more precise information will we be able to understand the contexts in which risk minimization strategies are being employed and therefore be better able to design prevention programs which are relevant to the lives of those in the target groups. Even in the absence of data to support a particularly high risk of HIV infection for homosexual men under 30 years old, it remains an important task for prevention work to not only establish safer sex norms in younger generations of gay men, but also to draw more attention to the necessity of maintaining risk-minimizing strategies over time.

The percentage of HIV-positive men swung between 10-12% for gay men surveyed in the five waves of the national Gay Press survey in West Germany conducted since 1987, without any indication of upward or downward trends. For West Germany, it appears that the most substantial behavioral changes among gay men took place from 1984-1986. New infections continue to take place among many men who show a high level of knowledge regarding means of transmission. The men are not becoming infected because of lack of information, but rather, in spite of their being well-informed.

This article was an attempt to determine to what extent deficient risk management in steady relationships is a cause for new infections. In another publication, the author has documented the particular vulnerability for HIV infection of working-class gay men in Germany (Bochow, 1997). This increased vulnerability is the result of working-class men's lack of integration into formal and informal gay networks, their lower level of education, their more limited opportunities for socializing, their greater degree of social isolation, and the necessity to hide their lives as gay men. These factors are causally interrelated. Improved risk management for couples and a more intensive outreach-oriented work in general are important steps for the future to reduce the infection rate for these groups to under the 10% mark.

REFERENCES

ACON, AIDS Council of New South Wales (1996). *Talk, test, test again, trust . . . together.* Sydney: AIDS Council of New South Wales.

AIDS/HIV: Quartalsbericht I (1997). 125. *Bericht des AIDS-Zentrums im Robert Koch-Institut über epidemiologische Daten.* Berlin.

Bochow, M. (1988). AIDS: Wie leben schwule Männer heute? Bericht über eine Befragung im Auftrag der Deutschen AIDS-Hilfe. *Berlin: AIDS-Forum D.A.H., II.*

Bochow, M. (1990). AIDS and gay men: Individual strategies and collective coping. *European Sociological Review* 6:181-188.

Bochow, M. (1994). Schwuler Sex und die Bedrohung durch AIDS. Reaktionen homosexueller Männer in Ost- und Westdeutschland. [Gay sex and the threat of AIDS–The reactions of gay men in Eastern and Western Germany]. *Berlin: AIDS-Forum D.A.H., XVI*:6-13.

Bochow, M. (1995). Data deserts and poverty of interpretation. Notes on deficiencies in Prevention-oriented research, taking gay men as an example. In D. Friedrich and W. Heckmann (Eds.), *AIDS in Europe–The Behavioral Aspect. Vol. 4: Determinants of Behavior Change.* Berlin: edition sigma, 249-257.

Bochow, M. (1997). Informationsstand und präventive Vorkehrungen im Hinblick auf AIDS bei homosexuellen Männern der Unterschicht. [The particular vulnerability of working class gay men to HIV infection and AIDS]. *Berlin: AIDS-Forum D.A.H., XXVI*:7-16.

Bochow, M., Chiarotti, F., Davies, P., Dubois-Arber, F., Dür, W., Fouchard, J., Gruet, F., McManus, T., Markert, S., Sandfort, T., Sasse, H., Schiltz, M.-A., Tielman, R., & Wasserfallen, F. (1994). Sexual behavior of gay and bisexual men in eight European countries. *AIDS Care*, 6(5):533-549.

Dannecker, M. (1990). *Homosexuelle Männer und AIDS. Eine sexualwissenschaftliche Studie zu Sexualverhalten und Lebensstil.* Berlin: Köln.

Dannecker, M. (1994). Im Liebesfall. *Aktuell: Das Magazin der Deutschen AIDS-Hilfe.* 7:16-20.

Dannecker, M. & Reiche, R. (1974). *Der gewöhnliche Homosexuelle. Eine soziologische Untersuchung über männliche Homosexuelle in der Bundesrepublik.* Frankfurt a. M.

Davies, P. M., Hickson, F. C. I., Weatherburn, O., & Hunt, A. J. (1993). *Sex, Gay Men and AIDS.* London: The Falmer Press.

de Zwart, O., van Kerkhof, M. P. N., & Sandfort, T. G. M. (1995). The structure and meaning of anal sex among gay men. In D. Friedrich and W. Heckmann (Eds.): AIDS in Europe. The Behavioral Aspect. Vol. 2: Risk Behavior and Its Determinants. Berlin, pp. 107-114.

Henriksson, B. (1995). Risk factor love. *Homosexuality, Sexual Interaction and HIV Prevention.* Göteborg: University of Göteborg.

Kippax, S. (1997). Social science and HIV prevention: A case study of gay community research. Keynote address presented at the 3rd International AIDS Impact Conference: *Biopsychosocial Aspects of HIV Infection.* Melbourne, Australia, 22-25 June.

Kippax, S., Connell, R.W., Dowsett, G.W., & Crawford, J. (1993). Sustaining safe sex: Gay Communities Respond to AIDS. London: The Falmer Press.

Moatti, J. P., Beltzer, N., & Dab, W. (1993). Les modèles d'analyse des comportements à risque face à l'infection à VIH: Une conception trop étroite de la rationalité. *Population*, 48(5): 1505-1534.

Pientka, L. (1994). Gesundheitliche Ungleichheit und das Lebensstilkonzept. A. Mielck (Ed.): *Krankheit und soziale Ungleichheit. Ergebnisse der sozialepidemiologischen Forschung in Deutschland.* Opladen: Leske und Budrich, 393-409.

Pollak, M. (1988). Les homosexuels et le SIDA. Sociologie d'une épidémie. Paris: Paris, Editions A. M. Métalié.

Schiltz, M.-A. (1993). Les homosexuels masculins face au SIDA: Enquêtes 1991-1992. Rapport de fin de contrat à l'ANRS. Paris: CAMS, CNRS.

Schiltz, M.-A. & Adam, P. (1995). Les homosexuels face au SIDA: Enquête 1993 sur les modes de vie et la gestion du risque VIH. Paris: CAMS, CERMES.

Gay Men and HIV: Community Responses and Personal Risks

Peter Keogh, BA
Susan Beardsell, PhD
Peter Davies, PhD
Ford Hickson, BSc
Peter Weatherburn, MSc

SUMMARY. This paper reports on the results of qualitative studies examining the personal experiences of sex and sexual negotiation for British gay men who are diagnosed HIV positive and those who know or presume themselves to be uninfected. These are contrasted with the results of a study of representations of HIV and AIDS within an international review of community health promotion literature aimed at gay men. The paper highlights the disparity between specific community responses to the epidemic as engendered in the cultural production of health promotion materials and the individual experience of HIV, suggesting a paradigm for a community response to the epidemic which reflects the personal experience of gay men both infected and uninfected. *[Article copies available for a fee from The Haworth Document Delivery Service: 1-800-342-9678. E-mail address: getinfo@haworthpressinc.com]*

Recent accounts of AIDS, both in the United States (Odets, 1994) and in the United Kingdom (Hickson et al., 1994), emphasize the formative role of HIV status on the personal experiences of gay men living through the epidemic. Whether one perceives or knows oneself to be HIV infected or uninfected will, to some extent, determine one's experiences of sex and sexual negotiation (Davies, Hickson, Weatherburn & Beardsell, 1995; Green, 1994; Keogh & Beardsell, 1997); love and friendship (Green, 1994; Keogh et al., 1995b; Odets, 1994); grief and mourning (Odets, 1994); and stigma (Green, 1994). Whilst the purpose of these studies are not to set up divisions between infected and uninfected gay men, they show how accepted gay community maxims such as *Positive or negative, it's the same for all* are simplistic and unhelpful.

The specific strength of these studies is that their analysis of the personal experiences and behaviors of gay men is informed by larger social realities, including interpersonal negotiations, gay community norms, historical relationships between stigma and disease, and gay identity. However, whilst most studies investigate subjective experience and individual behaviors, few attempt to analyze how gay men's experiences of AIDS and HIV are represented and constructed within specifically gay social discourses (such as the gay media, health promotion literature, club and bar advertisements). This paper is a comparison between the personal experiences of sex and sexual negotiation reported within mainly qualitative research into gay men (including both those diagnosed with HIV and those who know or presume themselves to be uninfected) and the representations of HIV and AIDS within community health promotion literature aimed at gay men.

The aim of this paper is to highlight the disparity between community responses to the epidemic on the one hand and individual experiences of HIV on the other. The focus, however, will be on sexual health and sexual negotiation. We will address the question of why it has taken nearly fifteen years for activist and/or community discourses on AIDS to incorporate the great differences between the lived experience of gay men diagnosed with HIV and that of gay men who know or believe themselves to be uninfected.

This paper is divided into two parts. The first part presents data from two studies of the personal experiences of sex and sexual functioning for gay men. One of these concentrates on the experiences of gay men diagnosed with HIV, whilst the other reports on the experiences of gay men who either know or presume themselves to be uninfected. The second part presents the results of an analysis of health promotion literature for gay men from several countries. Finally, a comparison is drawn in order to suggest a new paradigm for community response to the AIDS epidemic which both addresses the sexual health needs of gay men diagnosed with

HIV and the prevention needs of gay men who know or presume themselves to be uninfected.

There are difficulties with selecting appropriate terms to describe these two groups. We chose the terms *diagnosed with HIV* to cover those men who have received a positive test result for HIV. The phrase *know or presume themselves to be uninfected* describes both men who received a negative result the last time they were tested for HIV as well as those who have never been tested. Previous research carried out by SIGMA (Socio-sexual Investigation of Gay Men and AIDS) indicates that the majority of men in the United Kingdom who fit into the latter two groups currently assume themselves to be uninfected (Davies et al., 1993). We are therefore describing a very specific population.

A. PERSONAL EXPERIENCES OF HIV

For some time now, partner type has been established as one of the main correlates of condom use for anal intercourse between gay men (de Wit et al., 1994; Fitzpatrick, Boulton & Hart, 1990; Hunt et al., 1990). More recently, mainly qualitative research has shown that knowledge or perceptions of your own and your partner's HIV status is likely to affect condom use. That is, gay men are more likely to engage in unprotected anal intercourse with a partner whom they know or believe to be the same HIV status as themselves (Adib et al., 1991; Bosga et al., 1995; Doll et al., 1991; Hickson et al., 1992; Kippax et al., 1993; McLean et al., 1994; Ridge, Plummer & Minichiello, 1994; Schiltz & Adam, 1995). However, there is little research which investigates how this knowledge is gained or the circumstances in which decisions about condom use are made with different sexual partners. Moreover, the effect of this knowledge on other aspects of sexual and emotional functioning is still unclear. The following explores how knowledge of one's own and one's partner's HIV status affects sexual functioning for gay men diagnosed with HIV and those men who presume or know themselves to be uninfected.

Gay Men Diagnosed with HIV

Studies of gay men diagnosed with HIV tend to focus either on their contribution to the subsequent spread of the epidemic or on the impact of diagnosis and disease progression on psychological well-being (Green et al., 1992; Hedge et al., 1992). The differences in sexual functioning between this group and their undiagnosed counterparts were explored in a qualitative study conducted in the United Kingdom of gay men diagnosed with HIV (Keogh & Beardsell, 1997).

Ninety men were recruited through advertisements in the London gay press, at gay pubs and clubs, and at AIDS Service Organizations. The mean age of the sample was 31 years (range 21 to 54). Seventy-eight men were white European, eight were white non-European. Two men were African-Caribbean and one each was African and Asian. The mean number of years since an HIV-diagnosis was two-and-a-half with a range from three months to nine years. Eight had an AIDS diagnosis. The study concentrated on accounts of sexual encounters and accompanying reactions and emotions. We investigated, first, the impact of a positive diagnosis on sexual functioning and, secondly, the effect that knowledge of one's partner's HIV status has on sexual behavior.

The gay men in our study diagnosed with HIV tended to characterize their response to an HIV diagnosis in terms of either an increase or decrease in numbers of sexual partners. These responses could be arranged along a distinct continuum, the polar points of which are giving up sexual contact for a period (celibacy) and increasing the number of casual or anonymous sexual partners (sexual anonymity).

Recently HIV-diagnosed men characterized these reactions as emerging from a new and unpredicted anxiety about a perceived inability to negotiate sex now that they had a different HIV status. Two strong themes emerged relating to this anxiety. The first was a concern about disclosing one's HIV status to a sexual partner. The second was a concern about being solely responsible for the safety of a sexual encounter (that is, concerns about infecting sexual partners).

Respondents experienced their sexual partners' reactions to disclosing HIV status as problematic. First, they feared sexual rejection. Many had experienced this rejection, although the necessity to anticipate it was perceived as more damaging then actual rejection.

> ... And then, after all that chatting up and effort, having to anticipate the worst automatically, that this one might just be the one who will throw a real wobbly . . . to prepare yourself for that every time you have sex. I used to really enjoy cruising, you know, the chase, but this just wears you down.

Even when potential partners responded positively to a disclosure, this response was not always appropriate and could lead to an inordinate interest from sexual partners in the respondent's HIV disease. Respondents reported having to field inquiries about their general state of health, whether their friends had died, etc., in an encounter which was supposed to be enjoyable and sexual.

> You spend the whole evening talking about being sick and people dying. They don't seem to want to know anything about you, just your HIV. It's really rather depressing, like you're a freak or something.

Respondents experienced this as distressing, as an invasion of privacy, and as a substantial disincentive to disclose their diagnosis. If respondents did not disclose their HIV status to sexual partners, they felt that they had to take complete responsibility for the safety of the sexual encounter. The greatest fear in this context was accidentally infecting a partner, either through a faulty or broken condom or through oral sex (men were particularly worried about ejaculating in the mouth of their partners or the infectivity of their pre-ejaculate).

> What if the condom breaks and you don't notice? What do you tell him after if you haven't told him you're HIV already? There's no way to tell him then.

Respondents also worried about the effects of alcohol or drugs on their own or their partners' judgement. In addition, respondents were worried that a casual sexual encounter may result in a friendship or relationship, which many desired. However, they feared that the new relationship would be jeopardized when they subsequently disclosed their status.

> I'd like to think that I'll fall in love again, and you think, now, where does that happen? It happens between the sheets or over breakfast when you realize, *I really like him*. I won't let myself feel that because I know that as soon as I tell him, he'll run a mile.

This feeling of responsibility and secrecy was experienced by many as a barrier to intimacy and as something which made sexual encounters stressful. Thus, gay men diagnosed with HIV reported being in a *double bind*. If they disclosed their HIV status, they risked negative or inappropriate reactions which made sexual encounters problematic. If they did not disclose, they risked being found out or having to disclose after they had, perhaps, risked infecting a partner.

The key to these problems was the HIV positive men's concern with sexual negotiation, as opposed to a concern with sex itself. Consequently, an immediate coping reaction was to obviate the need for negotiation in a sexual encounter. Respondents who did not stop engaging in sex after a diagnosis reported a preference for having no emotional or social connection with their partners. For some, this meant a casual encounter. Others reported *not wanting to see the face* of their partners. These men did not desire to have unprotected sex with their partners; they merely did not want to have to verbally negotiate the sexual encounter.

Thus, the seemingly opposed reactions (celibacy and sexual anonymity) are different responses to the same problem, that is, a new and increased complexity in sexual negotiation. Men cope with this difficulty by either ceasing to have sex or having anonymous or casual sex (for which little or no verbal negotiation is necessary).

Most men subsequently developed a number of more successful strategies to improve their sexual negotiation. The first of these was re-learning the negotiation of sex. Many talked about acquiring new skills which they equated to learning how to "cruise" and "pick-up" when they first became sexually active. They learned who to tell:

> P1: Well you just sit there and listen to them for a while, you generally know whether or not to tell them.
>
> P2: How do you judge that?
>
> P1: Well if they're older for one, that helps, or if they haven't come out with anything that says, you know, 'I'm scared of AIDS' or if they talk about friends who have it. A good way is to bring AIDS into the conversation and see how they react, that's always a good one.

and when the best time was to tell:

> I always have to know them first and I always have to go to either my place or their place. It's not always that I decide to tell them . . . I do get to know whether to tell them in the place I meet them or I gauge whether to tell them when I get home; and with some people, I wait until we are going to start [sex] because you have to judge what some people want and you do get a reaction sometimes.

Prolonged contact with either formal or informal support networks of other gay men diagnosed with HIV was vital to the acquisition of these skills. The support of peers gained from these networks was also useful in enabling them to deal positively with rejection and off-loading the overwhelming sense of responsibility for the sexual safety of the encounter. By realizing that their partner was equally, but differently, responsible within the sexual encounter, men could begin to be more relaxed about sex. However, they still needed peer support to deal with mishaps, for example, with condom breakages.

Many men expressed a preference for sexual partners who were also diagnosed with HIV. This was for a variety of reasons. Not only did it reduce the difficulties associated with negotiating sex, but men also felt a certain emotional closeness and empathy for partners who were diagnosed with HIV which they did not necessarily feel for men who did not know their own status. The resulting sex was felt to be more satisfying, since they felt more at ease. Finally, some men concluded that they could have unprotected anal intercourse without any adverse health consequences.

Men Who Know or Assume Themselves to Be Uninfected

Another study conducted in the United Kingdom explored the circumstances under which a sample of gay men who knew or presumed themselves to be uninfected engaged in unprotected anal intercourse with both casual and regular partners (Davies et al., 1997). In this study, face-to-face, semi-structured life history interviews were conducted with 39 gay men recruited through a gay community newspaper. Ten men were interviewed from each of the age bands under 26, 26 to 35, and 36 to 45, and nine men over 45 were interviewed. Incidents of unprotected anal intercourse were either unplanned or planned.

Unplanned Incidents. These are incidents of unprotected anal intercourse which took place with no prior intention or planning, often the result of spur-of-the-moment decisions with a casual partner or perhaps in the context of a longer relationship. A number of circumstances were identified under which these suspensions of rational control occurred. Alcohol and recreational drugs were often implicated in these accounts, being away from home (for example on holiday), or returning from an extended period away from a regular partner.

The majority of the men regretted such incidents, characterizing them as wrong or unsafe, reporting resultant guilt and worry. This worry was generally associated with whether or not HIV had been passed on, most making post-hoc assessments of the likely HIV status of their sexual partners. Invariably, such assessments resulted in a decision that the sexual partner with whom unprotected sex occurred was most probably also not infected with HIV. Such assessments were made on the basis of the partner's age, looks, history, or behavior, amongst other things.

However, for men who had unprotected anal intercourse with men whom they suspected to be infected with HIV, a fatalism ensued where they presumed themselves to be infected. Often this served as a reason and/or excuse for condoms to be discarded entirely. However, this was the case mainly with regular partners.

Planned Incidents. Many of the men in the sample had recognized the limitations that the need to use condoms places on their sexual behavior and so proceeded to create situations in which they are able to be spontaneous, without guilt and fear (or at least with a reduction of the guilt and fear to acceptable levels). Thus, they are forging relationships and agreements within relationships that allow them to engage in unprotected anal intercourse while maintaining a regard for safety with respect to HIV transmission. The Australians have termed this "negotiated safety" (Kippax et al., 1993).

In most of these cases, couples arrive at the agreements through discussion. However, the type of discussion that is involved and the criteria that are used to make this decision vary. In some cases, it was an explicit discussion with a range of factors taken into account, such as sexual history, the relative ability of both partners to stick to agreements once they are made and to inform each other of transgressions, etc. However, for others, there was a heavy reliance on trust and love, with some men stating that it was a case of *putting your life on the line* for a partner. In these cases, most men felt that they were showing a clear-sighted acceptance of the real risks of living and loving in an epidemic.

Many respondents used HIV test results as an aid to their decision-making process, although the rigor with which test results are used varies. There are those who apply the results in an almost obsessive or ritualized manner, as well as those who incorporate testing into their decision-making in more considered ways. The explicitness in the use of test results in the negotiation process also varied. For some, it is based entirely on overt discussion. However, in many cases, there is a role for tacit knowledge regarding the likely HIV status of one's partners, either through results of a previous test or the discussion of past sexual history. In a few cases, however, discussion is at best vague and at worst non-existent.

There is clearly room in this process of negotiation for both deception and misunderstandings. This is reflected in a residual sense of unease reported by most men, regardless of the extent of the discussion with their partners. Thus, the decision to act strategically to avoid HIV transmission is patently not a once-and-for-all commitment, but one that requires constant monitoring and re-evaluation.

This research was useful in that it has shown something of the complexity–and often good sense–that underpins decisions to engage or not to engage in unprotected anal intercourse. Momentary lapses of judgement or of carefulness can and do result in incidents that the men involved later regret or feel guilty about. However, many instances of unprotected anal intercourse are premeditated. The range of information and analysis that underlies *negotiated safety* is varied, ranging from detailed, almost obsessive, discussion to the haphazard, collusive acceptance of unknown and uncertain risks.

When developing a personal response to HIV and sex, both men diagnosed with HIV and those who know or presume themselves to be uninfected depend crucially on an assessment of the relationship between their known or perceived HIV status and the larger socio-sexual world they inhabit. The range of sexual practices that individual gay men feel are acceptable in the midst of the epidemic (which could include using a condom, negotiated safety, cutting down on sexual partners, monogamy, not swallowing cum, not visiting saunas, etc.) are informed by an assessment of personal risk within a social network which is affected by (or infected with) a fatal sexually transmitted disease. The adoption of safer sex is a personal strategy. However, it is overwhelmingly within the social context of other gay men who may or may not be carrying the virus (my lover, my friend, the anonymous partner in the park, gay men generally). It is this social aspect that is of interest; namely, this reference of one's own vulnerability to being infected by another or one's own capacity to infect another.

The invention of safer sex by gay men is a continuing process which involves reacting to a major socio-sexual and medical problem in order to formulate a personal strategy. It is a community or group phenomenon, but crucially, it is dependent upon personal reactions. Both the problems which arise and the strategies developed to resolve them are dependent on one's own perceived or known HIV status and the presumed or known HIV status of one's sexual partners.

These individual responses to safer sex share further common characteristics. They are fundamentally dependent on personal–as opposed to collective–responsibility. Motivated largely by self-interest and the protection of the self, they emphasize the differences between people, as opposed to the similarities. The responses are contingent on circumstances, demanding a degree of mental dexterity. Moreover, they are not based on formulaic solutions to problems. Finally, the individual responses are not informed by any positive political ideology.

B. HEALTH PROMOTION MATERIALS

Having described processes informing the development of personal safer sex strategies, the remainder of this paper will specifically describe community responses to HIV and safer sex through an analysis of community-based health promotion and HIV prevention materials aimed at men. These materials were derived from three separate archives, one in the USA and two in the United Kingdom. They were produced between 1989 and 1994. The analysis covered 233 (mainly English-language) posters, postcards, and leaflets of which 39% originated in the United Kingdom, 19% were from Australia and 6% each from USA and Germany. The remaining materials originated in Belgium, Canada, Denmark, Finland, France, Ireland, Netherlands, Spain, Sweden and Switzerland. Eighty-one percent of the materials were posters, 12% were postcards and 7% were miscellaneous folded leaflets.

Although the vast majority of these materials (98%) mentioned HIV and AIDS, most (89%) did not address, mention, or represent gay men with HIV/AIDS (Keogh et al., 1995b). The materials reviewed yielded only 27 characters who could be unequivocally interpreted as being diagnosed with HIV and gay. Further analysis revealed three types of advertisements which perpetuated this exclusion.

The first were those which focused on diversity within the gay community (e.g., ethnic diversity; diversity of sexual practice and contexts; dress codes, etc.). However, most omitted listing difference in HIV status as another facet in the diversity of the gay male population.

The second type tended to address only those readers who assumed themselves to be uninfected. Often this was done in the form of advice: e.g., *Think about taking the test* or *There are two things you can do to protect yourself from the HIV virus....* This was also done by encouraging readers to remain uninfected. War imagery was common, *Know your enemy and fight it, don't let HIV in* (Postcard–United Kingdom).

The third type constructed an association between positive gay identity and the practice of safer sex. In other words, being a successful gay man was associated with condom use. Others established condom use as a means of identifying with other gay men and as a way of gaining acceptance as part of a gay community. Some went further in associating being a *good* gay man with being HIV negative, whilst one told the reader that he had *a responsibility to his community* to remain HIV negative.

Although HIV itself appears almost universally within health promotion materials for gay men, those diagnosed with HIV are all but invisible. The approaches outlined above not only fail to affirm HIV-positive identity but suggest that a positive test result excludes the individual from an active role within a wider gay community. Moreover, there is little in these materials to indicate the extent to which HIV has actually affected both the general population of gay men as well as the infected gay men living within that population.

The effect of this *depersonalization* of gay men diagnosed with HIV is enhanced by a common tendency of health promotion materials to talk almost exclusively of protecting oneself from the virus whilst stopping short of saying exactly where the source of this possible infection would be (from another gay man's body). Health promotion specialists are clearly concerned not to be seen as demonizing gay men diagnosed with HIV as *infecting agents* or *reservoirs of infection*. However, this approach can have the added effect of never encouraging a man who is at present uninfected to think of his own HIV prevention in personal terms, that is, that any of his sexual partners may be infected with HIV.

Materials which did represent gay men diagnosed with HIV/AIDS tended to do so in two ways. First, they encouraged a specific community response to HIV based on socio-sexual identity:

> Our community is diverse. . . . We all share being gay and we share the effects that HIV has on our community, our friends, our partners, ourselves. Our love–gay love–will help us survive. Our community is stronger than ever. Fight AIDS, always have safe sex. . . . (Poster–Australia)

Secondly, they sought to give the same sexual health advice to gay men, regardless of their HIV status. The following is written with no reference to re-infection with HIV:

> The guidelines for safer sex are the same if you're HIV-positive, negative or don't know. Fucking is by far the biggest risk in sex. (Postcard–United Kingdom)

However, by failing to explain what the real danger is (becoming infected) and by attempting to minimize or de-emphasize the differences between gay men diagnosed with HIV and gay men who know or presume themselves to be uninfected, these leaflets address practically none of the sexual health and prevention needs of either constituency (on the one hand, the uninfected man's need to protect himself from infection, and on the other hand, the diagnosed man's needs to protect himself from the adverse health and social consequences of his infection and not to infect others).

Analysis of these and the other advertisements in the review yielded a number of clear characteristics of health promotion materials. Materials included in this sample tended not to represent gay men diagnosed with HIV. They speak about the dangers of HIV to gay men who presume or know themselves to be uninfected, but consistently ignore the source of infection (the body of a gay man who is infected). Many mentioned gay men diagnosed with HIV, but attempted to reduce the differences between this group and gay men who are uninfected, thus addressing the needs of both constituencies inadequately. Finally, many tended to foster "community" responses to HIV by encouraging a gay community to care for and identify with its positive members, characterizing the use of a condom as a way of expressing that identification. The tiny percentage of resources that do address the needs of gay men diagnosed with HIV rarely represent or advise on sexual health issues or needs.

The analysis revealed a central discourse around HIV and gay men diagnosed with HIV. HIV is characterized as a disembodied threat to a community, which can be defeated through community ties of solidarity. This discourse has two levels. The first assumes that everyone within that community is uninfected at present. This implies that the action of the virus is to make people disappear (or die, although, interestingly, death is never mentioned), as opposed to living within that community in an infected state. The second is one which concedes that people who become infected with the virus do indeed live on and remain sexually active for a period. However, the danger for an uninfected man of having unprotected sex with an infected man is never explicitly stated. That is, that an infected gay man has within his body a virus that can be transmitted through unprotected sex to the body of an uninfected gay man. Therefore, although within this second discourse, condom use is stressed, the reason for using a condom (as a barrier to the transmission of HIV from one body to another) is never stated. Instead, community is again stressed so that the act of wearing a condom is one which expresses solidarity with one's fellow gay men, be they infected or not. The act of wearing a condom becomes disassociated with the avoidance of disease. Therefore, the sexual health needs of both groups (gay men diagnosed with HIV and those who presume or know themselves to be uninfected) are neither reflected nor addressed within this literature. Finally and crucially, the materials diverge greatly from the experiences of individual gay men.

There is clearly a gulf in personal responses to HIV and safer sex and how these responses are represented in health promotion discourses which seek to engender collective or community response. These differences may be accounted for in an analysis of social science research in the epidemic. Some studies have shown positive correlations between levels of community attachment and reductions in unsafe sex (Kippax, Crawford & Connell, 1992). However, there are a number of ways in which this correlation can be interpreted, and different interpretations may lead to radically different health promotion strategies. Two possible interpretations are examined here. The first is one that we are generally familiar with. In this interpretation, community attachment leads to high self-esteem and therefore to a greater desire to protect oneself. The resulting HIV prevention strategy is clear:

promote community attachment and HIV prevention through political identity and ties of gay solidarity (Kippax et al., 1993).

The alternative interpretation is as follows. It is precisely men who are attached to a gay community who see themselves as most at risk. The increased perception of personal risk that came with gay identity led to reductions in unprotected sex. This theory calls for educational strategies which support personal responsibility and encourage communication between gay men, thereby encouraging gay men to explore how differences in HIV status affect sexual, emotional and social interaction. This second interpretation is attractive, as it doesn't idealize individual gay men or the community in which they live; it recognizes the presence of an epidemic and of gay men diagnosed with HIV as sexually active. It does not provide simplistic or formulaic solutions to complex social, emotional and sexual problems and, finally, it encourages gay men to make rational decisions based on their personal assessment of risk.

The former interpretation (the *community* discourse surrounding HIV and gay men diagnosed with HIV) radically distorts the reality of gay men's experiences and decision-making in relation to HIV and safer sex. We have seen how this process is damaging because it fails to address the sexual health needs of both gay men diagnosed with HIV and men who know or presume themselves to be uninfected. We can also see the origin of the gulf of lived experience between these two groups as eclipsed by simplistic chants such as *Positive and negative, it's the same for all*, and, *Positive or negative, a condom protects us all*. The reality is clearly different. It is the successful and creative assessment of personal risk and deciding on an appropriate risk reduction strategy (which may or may not involve the use of a condom) that protects a man who knows himself to be uninfected from contracting the virus and a man diagnosed with HIV from becoming re-infected or from passing on the virus. These are very different risks. In addition, this specific community response to HIV has more damaging effects. It may stifle individual creative thought in relation to HIV, de-valuing gay men's vital experience and inventive expertise in relation to formulating successful strategies around risk assessment and avoidance. It discourages individual responsibility for not contracting or passing on the virus. It may discourage community solidarity where it is needed most, that is, in the form of a real understanding and empathy on the part of gay men who know or presume themselves to be uninfected for the lives of men who are diagnosed with HIV. Finally, by failing to represent the reality of living with HIV, in both it's positive and negative aspects, it fails to represent what HIV negative men need to avoid when they are practicing safer sex (that is, it fails to give them a reason to practice safer sex other than being a *good* gay man).

CONCLUSION

The promotion of safer sex within gay communities cannot, therefore, be about slogans or simplistic solutions to complex problems. Appealing to gay men as members of a gay community and giving them *support* to practice safer sex is insufficient. This approach is entirely counter-intuitive to all of our notions of risk and its management. Gay men can be supported to feel good about themselves as gay men; however, support alone does not help gay men to practice safer sex. Instead, gay men should be appealed to as individuals first, individuals who every day make sexual choices in the management of their personal risk.

REFERENCES

Adib, S. M., Joseph, J. G., Ostrow, D. G., Tal, M., & Schwartz, S. A. (1991). Relapse in sexual behavior among homosexual men: A 2-year follow-up from the Chicago MACS/CCS. *AIDS*, 5(6): 757-60.

Bosga, M. B., de Wit, J. B., de-Vroome, E. M., Houweling, H., Schop, W., & Sandfort, T. G. (1995). Differences in perception of risk for HIV infection with steady and non-steady partners among homosexual men. *AIDS Education and Prevention*, 7(2): 103-15.

Davies, P. M., Hickson, F. C. I., Weatherburn, P., & Hunt, A. J. (1993). *Gay Men, Sex and AIDS*. London: The Falmer Press.

Davies, P. M., Hickson, F., Weatherburn, P., & Beardsell, S. (1995). The maintenance of safer sexual behavior among gay and bisexual men in the United Kingdom: A report to the Health Education Authority (unpublished report). London: SIGMA Research.

de Wit, J. B., Teunis, N., van Griensven, G. J., & Sandfort, T. G. (1994). Behavioral risk-reduction strategies to prevent HIV infection among homosexual men: A grounded theory approach. *AIDS Education and Prevention*, 6(6): 493-505.

Doll, L. S., Byers, R. H., Bolan, G., Douglas, J. M., Jr., Moss, P. M., Weller, P. D., Joy, D., Bartholow, B. N., & Harrison, J. S. (1991). Homosexual men who engage in high-risk sexual behavior. A multicenter comparison. *Sexually Transmitted Diseases*, 18(3): 170-5.

Fitzpatrick, R., Boulton, M., & Hart, G. (1990). Variation in sexual behavior in gay men. In P. Aggleton, P. M. Davies, & G. Hart (Eds.), *AIDS: Individual, Cultural and Policy Dimensions*. London: Falmer, 121-33.

Green, G. (1994). Positive sex: Sexual relationships following an HIV positive diagnosis. In P. Aggleton, P. Davies, & G. Hart (Eds.), *AIDS: Foundations for the Future*. London: Taylor & Francis.

Green, J., Henderson, F., Tyrer, P., & Hedge, B. (1992). Subjective quality of life in persons with HIV disease. Poster Presentation for *VIII International Conference on AIDS*, 19-24 July, Amsterdam, PO-B-3565.

Hedge, B., Slaughter, J., Flynn, R., & Green, J. (1992). Coping with HIV disease: Successful attributes and strategies. Poster Presentation for *VIII International Conference on AIDS*, 19-24 July, Amsterdam, PO-B-1691.

Hickson, F. C., Davies, P. M., Hunt, A. J., Weatherburn, P., McManus, T. J., & Coxon, A. P. M. (1992). Maintenance of open gay relationships: Some strategies for protection against HIV. *AIDS Care*, 4(4): 409-19.

Hickson, F., Weatherburn, P., Davies, P. M., Hunt, A. J., Coxon, A. P. M., & McManus, T. J. (1992). Why gay men engage in anal intercourse. Poster presentation for *VIII International Conference on AIDS*, 19-24 July, Amsterdam, PO-D-5185.

Hickson, F. C. I., Weatherburn, P., Keogh, P., & Davies, P. (1994). Perceptions of partners' status and unprotected anal intercourse (UAI) among gay men. Oral presentation for the *2nd International Conference on Biopsychosocial Aspects of HIV Infection*, Brighton, United Kingdom, 7-10 July.

Hunt, A. J., Christofinis, G., Coxon, A. P. M., Davies, P. M., & McManus, T. J. (1990). Sero-prevalence of HIV-1 infection in a cohort of homosexually active men. *Genitourinary Medicine*, 66: 423-7.

Keogh, P., Beardsell, S., Hickson, F. C. I., & Reid, D. S. (1995a). *The Sexual Health Needs of HIV Positive Gay and Bisexual Men*. London: Camden Social Service/Camden & Islington Community Health Services NHS Trust.

Keogh, P., Beardsell, S., Hickson, F., Reid, D., & Stephens, M. (1995b). *The Support and Resource Needs of Gay Men with HIV/AIDS, Their Partners and Carers*. A report to the Terrence Higgins Trust (unpublished report). London: SIGMA Research.

Keogh P. & Beardsell, S. (1997). Sexual negotiation strategies of HIV-positive gay men: A qualitative approach. In P. Aggleton, P. Davies & G. Hart (Eds.), *AIDS: Activism and Alliances*. London: Taylor & Francis.

Kippax, S., Crawford, J., & Connell, R. (1992). The importance of the gay community in the prevention of HIV transmission: A study of Australian men who have sex with men. In P. Aggleton, P. Davies, & G. Hart (Eds.), *AIDS: Rights, Risks & Reasons*. London: Falmer Press.

Kippax, S., Crawford, J., Davis, M., Rodden, P., & Dowsett, G. (1993). Sustaining safe sex: A longitudinal study of a sample of homosexual men. *AIDS*, 7(2): 257-63.

McClean, J., Bouton, M., Brookes, M., Lakhani, D., Fitzpatrick, R., Dawson, J., McKechnie, R., & Hart, G. (1994). Regular partners and risky behavior: Why do gay men have unprotected intercourse? *AIDS Care*, 6(3): 331-41.

Odets, W. (1994). AIDS education and harm reduction for gay men: Psychological approaches for the 21st Century. *AIDS and Public Policy Journal*, 9: 1-18.

Ridge, D. T., Plummer, D. C., & Minichiello, V. (1994). Knowledge and practice of sexual safety in Melbourne gay men in the nineties. *Australian Journal of Public Health*, 18(3): 319-25.

Schiltz, M. A., & Adam, P. (1995). Reputedly effective risk reduction strategies and gay men. In P. Aggleton, P. M. Davies, & G. Hart (Eds.), *AIDS: Safety, Sexuality and Risk*. London: Falmer, 1-19.

In This Together: The Limits of Prevention Based on Self-Interest and the Role of Altruism in HIV Safety

David Nimmons, BA

SUMMARY. Both epidemiologically and psychologically, the reigning self-interest paradigm of HIV prevention is growing increasingly obsolete, which will likely only increase with wider use of combination therapies. While self-interest notions form the core of most American HIV prevention theory and practice, data indicate that self-interest models increasingly fail both negative and positive gay men. There is an urgent need for broader, more emotionally-resonant prevention concepts. Diverse, consistent, and significant data on behaviors including condom use, partner choice, volunteerism, and caretaking imply that values of altruism and other-centered motivators may play central, strong roles in gay men's HIV safety decisions. Values of "prevention altruism" remain little understood, researched, or appreciated. Data show that sexual risk is inherently dyadic, gay men's risk is increasingly relational, and a clear majority of gay men consistently manage sexual risk. Yet we understand little of the values of men who are largely safe, instead of those most risky, and less about how their values of nurturance and caretaking, ethics, hopes for collective survival, or relations with friends and community help support them in staying safe. A wide range of implications of prevention altruism are suggested and diverse research directions proposed to define a new domain of "prevention caretaking." *[Article copies available for a fee from The Haworth Document Delivery Service: 1-800-342-9678. E-mail address: getinfo@haworthpressinc.com]*

In the last fifteen years the dominant paradigm for HIV prevention among American gay men has been overwhelmingly characterized by an ethic of every man for himself. Based on a rudimentary analysis of self-interest, HIV prevention programs have largely urged at-risk gay men to safeguard their own health. Under this quintessentially consumerist paradigm, the goal of safer sex has been maximizing the self-interest of the two, or more, parties involved. By implication, the interest of the man on the other end of the condom has differed from one's own. Accordingly, HIV prevention has alternatively emphasized self-protection through information, disclosure, and the skills of sexual negotiation before the deal is consummated. In this form of erotic capitalism, the rule has been: *Let the buyer beware.* Implicitly, each man has been in it alone.

In this model of *me-first* prevention, both the responsibility and the concern for staying uninfected largely rests with the individual. It is one's own responsibility to stay safe, and one does so for oneself. Often, the roles of positive and negative men–as discussed among prevention workers, within the gay community, and within the popular press–are depicted so as to place responsibility for sexual safety primarily in the hands of one partner (or class of partners, such as infected men). In public discourse, through incantations of *positive men should* . . . and *negative men must* . . ., the burden is largely placed on the individual to look out for number one. Ironically, such views seem to overlook the fact that HIV transmission is intrinsically a dyadic act, occurring during the most intimate of shared moments, between actors embedded in a web of social relationships.

THE LIMITS OF SELF-INTEREST

Mounting data suggest that this stark self-interest paradigm is growing increasingly obsolete in at least two demonstrable ways. The most obvious is epidemiological. As rates of seroprevalence rise in a population, the proportion of men with a self-interest in remaining uninfected shrinks. In American epicenters like New York and San Francisco, HIV seroprevalence rates have been estimated over the years to range from one-third to more than 50% (Hoover et al., 1991; Torrian & Weisfuse, 1996; Winkelstein et al., 1987). In such communities, as many as one-in-two or one-in-three of the men seeking sexual partners on a given evening are already infected and, therefore, have minimal self-interest in avoiding HIV infection by practicing safer sex. Prevention programs that exhort a population with such a high seroprevalence to avoid infection are the public health equivalent of reminding the occupants of a burning house not to play with matches. Unless we find another way to speak to HIV-infected men, appeals that are predicated on one's self-interest in remaining uninfected are simply irrelevant. Although this problem may be most evident in epicenters with relatively high infection rates, the difficulty in appealing to infected men is similar elsewhere, regardless of the scope of the local epidemic.

The second problem with the self-interest paradigm is qualitatively different. Whereas the first deals with infected men and epidemiological realities, the second has to do with both positive and negative men and the psychological realities of sexual relationships. After a decade and a half of hearing prevention framed as a formidable personal task, gay men now consistently report that their safety challenges have as much to do with their relationships as with them as individuals (Hays and Kegeles, 1996; Hunt et al., 1992; McLean et al., 1994; Stall et al., 1990).

Gay men–regardless of their serostatus–are telling HIV prevention researchers and educators what pregnant adolescents have long said: *Unprotected sex feels like an act of intimacy and connection* (Davies et al., 1993; Kelly et al., 1991; Prieur, 1990). For HIV positive and negative men alike, unprotected sex has become a way to feel less alone, less disconnected, and less isolated, as well as a way to demonstrate love, trust, and faithfulness (Boulton et al., 1995; Gold et al., 1991). The leitmotif of risk is one of merging, of cleaving to, of bonding. The decision to have sex without a condom takes place in a relational context. There is scarcely a more consistent finding among gay men–from Australia to Amsterdam–than the clearly documented pattern that risk occurs most often in intimate relationships (Green, 1996; Hays, Kegeles, & Coates, 1990; Hoff et al., 1996; McLean et al., 1994).

This situation reveals the limits of the *every man for himself* philosophy. Gay men clearly seek to balance affiliative needs for affection and intimacy with a desire to avoid transmitting or being infected with HIV. Prevention strategies such as negotiated safety seek to recognize explicitly this difficulty, supporting men in performing a more nuanced prevention calculus, taking into account the risks of unprotected sex and the rewards of intimacy and connection under highly-constrained circumstances (Kippax et al., 1997). The overwhelming reliance on a model which focuses on the individual making the decision to stay safe ignores what gay men are telling us about the nature of their relationships. Given the importance of the relational context for risk-taking, the relentless placing of responsibility for safety on the shoulders of each individual may have the paradoxical effect of increasing the sense of alienation, disconnection and loneliness which may drive men to risky behaviors in the first place.

There is an urgent need for prevention work to elaborate a range of broader, more emotionally resonant prevention concepts. We are called to embrace and articulate credible motivators which move beyond the sole focus on individual self-preservation. If we do not, HIV prevention risks drifting into increasing irrelevance.

CONSIDERING THE EVIDENCE FOR HIV PREVENTION ALTRUISM

A wide range of beliefs, ideals, and values have gone largely untapped in HIV prevention practice. These include values beyond self-interest which play a role in gay men's sexual safety decisions. Central to these is a deeper recognition of what might be termed *prevention altruism.*

Where altruism is generally used in a broad sense to mean concern for others' welfare–in contrast to pure self-interest or egoism–prevention altruism is being defined here to include the values, motivations, and practices of caretaking in one's sexual behavior which arise out of a concern for others. In its most narrow sense, this means taking care that one's sexual partners do not become infected by disease. More broadly, it may include concern for the effects which being infected could have on others– from one's family or friends to a larger group, such as the gay community. Whether a man uses condoms to protect his evening's trick or out of devotion to his long-term lover; whether he wants to spare his mother the pain of his illness and death or express a commitment not to place more members of the gay community in danger–he is moved by values of prevention altruism, a concern for others' well-being which directly affects his sexual behavior.

Such altruism is extremely well-attested in the literature, if we but look. It is most strikingly seen in the many studies over the last decade which have shown greater risk reduction among seropositive men than among HIV-untested or seronegative men. For example, McCusker (1988) found that men who knew they were infected were far less likely to continue practicing unprotected insertive anal sex than positive men who did not know their status (33% versus 80%). The positive men who knew their status were also less likely than uninfected men to continue practicing unprotected insertive anal intercourse. Van Griensven et al. (1989) found that infected men were more likely to use condoms during insertive anal intercourse with both steady and non-steady partners than were seronegative men. In all, more than a dozen studies have found seropositive men to be more likely than seronegative or untested men to use condoms with steady or casual partners (Coates et al., 1989; Dawson et al., 1991; Farthing et al., 1987; Frazer et al., 1988; Fox et al., 1987; Higgins et al., 1991; McKusick et al., 1990).

The implications of repeated findings of high levels of condom use among a majority of HIV-positive men are striking in their implications (Coates et al., 1988; Hoff et al., 1996; Schechter et al., 1988; Tindall et al., 1989; Voigt et al., 1992). Such findings pose a clear challenge to conventional assumptions of simple self-interest. We cannot help but ask: Who exactly are positive men wearing condoms for? And why? What might be going on that motivates such consistent majorities of infected men to undertake an act which has such important social and emotional cost and to do so with seemingly far less apparent benefit? How are these men defining *self-interest*, and where does it intersect with *other-interest*?

Given recent developments in viral typing and testing, it might be argued that HIV positive men's self-interest concerning re-infection is the primary motive here. While that may be true in some cases, at least two sets of data should give pause to such an interpretation. First, had large numbers of positive men been primarily motivated by concerns about re-infection, one would expect them to have protected sex regardless of their partners' serostatus. Yet clear and consistent data indicate far lower rates of condom use among infected men with their seroconcordant partners than with seronegatives (Kippax et al., 1993; Exner et al., 1992; Sacco et al., 1996). The well-attested asymmetry in risk behavior with known seroconcordant partners suggests that self-protective concerns cannot solely–or even largely–explain the patterns of condom use documented in the clear majority of infected men. Secondly, in America at least, contemporary concerns about re-infection, deriving from recent developments in viral testing and typing technology, are a relatively recent phenomenon, attested in the scientific literature only in the last few years (Root-Bernstein, 1993) and in the popular literature far more recently (Schoofs, 1997). There are little data to suggest that re-infection was a widespread concern among large numbers of infected men at the time of the studies cited here.

Both patterns of lower levels of unprotected anal sex in serodiscordant couples (Marks, 1994; Remien, 1995) as well as partner selection data suggesting that HIV-positive men prefer positive partners (Marks, 1994; Service & Blowers, 1995) raise similar issues. Obviously, infected men may have many reasons to prefer infected partners, for example, shared bonds of life experience, treatment concerns, being more at ease with AIDS, etc. But concerns over infecting a partner are so commonly expressed and so deeply felt in many HIV positive men's narratives, that a larger range of values and motivations merits closer examination and understanding.

Rather than suggesting that infected men do not care, such sexual behavior findings imply that large numbers of these men indeed behave as though they care deeply, but about something larger than their self-interest. Perhaps, for an HIV-infected man, using a condom is less an act of self-interest than one of ethics. It may best be understood as an act of altruism. It is at least plausible that the HIV prevention strategies of many gay men reflect a central–largely unrecognized–role of prevention altruism at work in this community.

If altruism plays an important role in the values of gay men, one would expect to see it evidenced in realms beyond sexual behavior. In fact, significant data indicate that this is precisely the case. To see striking and suggestive evidence that altruistic motivators function robustly among gay men, one need only peruse the literature on partner selection, HIV disclosure, caretaking, volunteerism, or vaccine trials. Unprecedented community-wide HIV-related caregiving (Turner, Catania, & Gagnon, 1994), the pioneering of buddy systems and informal care partner networks, and widespread community participation in volunteer activities (Snyder & Omoto, 1994) reflect community values of acting on behalf of others. National vaccine trial data reveal high levels of other-directed motivators among this population for participation in research protocols (Hays et al., 1996).

A variety of such evidence, both in the sexual realm and beyond, reflect what community-based HIV prevention workers and gay men have long known. Properly understood, these data strongly suggest that other-focused concerns already operate as consistent, strong values among gay men, including being a part of their HIV risk-management strategies. In point of fact, gay men are saving each others' lives every night of the week, and have been doing so for the better part of two decades–not, to be sure, each and every time. But protecting each other appears to be a fairly consistent and normative practice in the majority of men surveyed in many core gay communities, judging by reported patterns of condom use among those reached by the first generation of prevention activity (Binson et al., 1995; Bochow et al., 1994; Hunt et al., 1993; Voigt et al., 1992).

These findings are consistent enough that we might well ask ourselves some simple questions: Why do dominant prevention paradigms largely ignore this set of altruistic values, beliefs, and motives? Why have we such difficulty transcending truisms of self-interest? Why does the academic literature on determinants of risk dwarf the literature on determinants of safety? Why have we spent so much more time on exploring the minority of men who are consistently unsafe than on the majority of men who by-and-large succeed in consistently avoiding risk?

In aggregate, much HIV prevention literature presents a fairly consistent picture: A significant body of studies, from a variety of nations, suggest that in the range of 60% to 70% of gay men surveyed appear to be practicing some form of sexual safety the majority of the time (Binson et al., 1995; Bochow, 1994; Hunt, 1993; Meyer & Dean, 1995; Myers, 1996; Ridge et al., 1994; Roffman et al., 1995). In cases where researchers can factor in data on serostatus of partners, the numbers climb even further (Hoff, 1996; Kippax, 1993; Remien, 1995). While we cannot discount higher levels of risk observed in specific studies and specific groups (most notably younger men, men of color, and prevention-naïve gay men), the basic trend is eminently clear: most gay men, most of the time, engage in some form of risk-management. The point is not that their strategies are necessarily foolproof, airtight, and 100% consistent, but rather, that as HIV prevention theorists we would do well to interrogate and better understand the values which underlie and motivate such a clear and widespread pattern of protective choices. One of those values may be altruism.

Perhaps the reason for the neglect of other-centered motives in prevention is that altruism is often viewed, at best, as being hopelessly impractical or, at worst, dangerously naïve. One wonders how many HIV prevention programs, for example, explore the ways infected men may find personal meaning in their disrupted lives by keeping other men alive. One is hard pressed to cite interventions which forthrightly engage the ways that keeping another man uninfected is a caring and humane act. In the face of what experts have characterized as *the most profound behavioral changes ever recorded in the history of public health* (Stall et al., 1988), we have failed to grasp what these populations are telling us in their actions, as seen across a wide range of behaviors.

It would be a sad irony indeed were historians of science and public health to write that we had evidence of some of the finest and most noble human values being exhibited by large numbers of people every day, yet HIV prevention theory and practice was unable to assimilate the lessons these communities offered. The task before us, in the quest for new and more emotionally resonant prevention paradigms, is to investigate what potential may lie in tapping additional powerful motivations currently manifest among gay men, both infected and uninfected. (Although the current discussion focuses on the communal practices of gay men, there is no a priori reason to believe that prevention altruism could not prove a similarly fruitful area of investigation in other at-risk populations.)

TESTING AND APPLYING HIV PREVENTION ALTRUISM

Clearly, formative research is necessary to test ideas of prevention altruism and to explore the paths they may open toward a broader set of motivators to HIV safety. A number of research and intervention questions may be delineated from this model, including:

- Can we identify for what men, in what ways, and in what circumstances, values pertaining to protecting others come into play to reduce HIV risk?
- How might prevention work best acknowledge the depth of altruism, caretaking, and nurturing which gay men currently engage in? How might such a recognition change how gay men act in terms of risk behavior?
- Do positive and negative men identify reciprocal roles and interests in keeping men uninfected?
- Do gay men conceive of safer sex as a form of caretaking or as saving another man's life? Are there covenants of caring that infected and uninfected gay men make with each other?
- How do motives for safety differ according to HIV status?
- Are there ways that protected sex provides a source of personal meaning, pride, or power for infected or uninfected men?
- Do notions of caretaking apply to the uninfected as well as to the infected?
- Do values underlying protected sexual practice in any way resemble values involved in caretaking of the sick?
- Do some gay men experience protected sex as a political act?
- Is protecting the next generation of gay men important to older generations of men?
- In what ways do our extended social relationships of family and friends affect sexual safety decisions? Is sexual safety linked to feelings about taking care of or caring for individuals beyond one's self and sexual partner?
- Do gay men who feel any of these things find other men with whom they can share their feelings and values?
- Are there cultural, geographic, age- or ethnicity-related effects in how prevention altruism is experienced, understood, or enacted?

- What range of interventions might speak to these motivators? How can messages, campaigns, and other interventions better reflect values that transcend self-interest?
- Might a richer understanding of prevention altruism help broaden our reliance on public health models? In particular, are lessons from social change traditions–e.g., feminism, civil rights, community empowerment and pedagogy–applicable to HIV prevention?

Broadening the dominant self-interest paradigm also requires that we move beyond the individual level of analysis to dyadic and communal levels, so as to better address the relational issues which gay men tell us impede their safety. Axiomatically, infection takes two; therefore, it behooves us all to stop assigning the motivation and onus for safer sex to one or the other partner. An approach integrally tied to issues of altruism and shared responsibility might better reflect the dyadic nature of risk as well as the risk reduction concerns gay men actually have. A better understanding of values of affection, intimacy, caretaking, and community offer alternatives to the atomization and isolation which men report increasingly threatens their ability to stay safe.

In the era of combination therapies, we are urgently challenged to forge a discourse and to create interventions which speak to the common needs of uninfected and infected people. Such interventions might require us to better acknowledge the common stakes, shared values, and mutual interests, and to affirm the myriad ways gay men find meaning in taking care of each other. This need not lead to a set of undifferentiated interventions; the stakes for infected and uninfected differ radically. But it would require us to clarify the ways men share such stakes across serostatus. It would also challenge us to give voice to the covenants gay men make with and for each other and to explore the values that inspire and sustain them. A clearer recognition of prevention altruism offers one way to do that.

Obviously, it is not the case that everything that is not self-interest is altruism; nor that these two tendencies are mutually exclusive. Humans are complicated creatures, and in any given individual at any given time, both tendencies may co-occur and even magnify each other. But it would seem inarguable that prevention thinkers need to more fully understand the range of ways men find meaning in supporting and maintaining sexual safety.

CONCLUSION

Across several domains, provocative data suggest that values of altruism and caretaking reflect a robust, if unrecognized, community norm among many gay men. A more explicit recognition of prevention altruism promises to open fundamentally new ground in prevention theory and practice. It may help lay the conceptual groundwork for a new generation of interventions and prevention programs. Perhaps it will help us point the way to developing notions of a shared collective stake in keeping people uninfected.

It remains an open question whether prevention workers can support at-risk communities in an ethos of supporting and caring for each other. In the meantime, gay men are showing us what they care about. It is up to us to listen.

REFERENCES

Binson, D., Michaels, S., Stall, R., Coates, T., Gagnon, J., & Catania, J. (1995). Prevalence and social distribution of men who have sex with men: United States and its urban centers. *Journal of Sex Research, 32*(3):245-254.

Bochow, M., Chiarotti, F., Davies, P., Dubois-Arber, F., Dur, W., Fouchard, J., Gruet, F., McManus, T., Markert, S., Sandfort, T., Sasse, H., Schiltz, M.-A., & Tielfallen, F. (1994). Sexual behavior of gay & bisexual men in eight European countries. *AIDS Care, 6*(4):533-549.

Boulton, M., McLean, J., Fitzpatrick, R., & Hart, G. (1995). Gay men's accounts of unsafe sex. *AIDS Care, 7*(5):619-30.

Coates, T. J., Morin, S. F., & McKusick, L. (1987). Behavioral consequences of AIDS antibody testing among gay men [letter]. *Journal of the American Medical Association, 258*:1889.

Coates, T. J., Stall, R. D., Kegeles, S. M., Lo, B., Morin, S., & McKusick, L. (1988). AIDS antibody testing: Will it stop the AIDS epidemic? Will it help people infected with HIV? *American Psychologist, 43*:859-864.

Davies, P. M., Hickson, F. C. I., Weatherburn, P., Hunt, A. J. (1993). *Sex, Gay Men, & AIDS*. London: Falmer Press.

Dawson, J., Fitzpatrick, R., McLean, J., Hart, G., & Boulton, M. (1991). The HIV test and sexual behaviour in a sample of homosexually active men. *Social Science Medicine, 32*:683-688.

Exner, T., Meyer-Bahlberg, H. F., & Erhardt, A. A. (1992, July). Effects of individual and partner sero-status on condom use. International Conference on AIDS; D450 (abstract no. PoD5381).

Farthing, C. F., Jessen, W., Taylor, H. L., Lawrence, A. G., & Gazzard, B. G. (1987, June). The HIV antibody test: Influence on behavior of homosexual men. Paper presented at the Third International Conference on AIDS, Washington, DC.

Fox, R., Odaka, N. J., Brookmeyer R., & Polk, B. F. (1987). Effect of HIV antibody disclosure on subsequent sexual activity in homosexual men. *AIDS, 1*:241-246.

Fox, R., Ostrow, D., Valdisseri, R., VanRaden, B., & Polk, B. F. (1987, June).

Changes in sexual activities among participants in the Multi-Center AIDS Cohort Study. Paper presented at the Third International Conference on AIDS, Washington, DC.

Frazer, I. H., McCamish, M., Hay, I., & North, P. (1988). Influence of human immunodeficiency virus antibody testing on sexual behaviour in a "high-risk" population from a "low-risk" city. *Medical Journal of Australia, 149*:365-368.

Gold, R., Skinner, M., Grant, P., & Plummer, D. (1991). Situational factors and thought processes associated with unprotected intercourse in gay men. *Psychology and Health, 5*:259-278.

Green, J. (1996, September 15). Flirting with Suicide. *New York Times Magazine*, 38-85.

Hays, R. & Kegeles, S. (1996, February 11-15). Factors related to willingness of young gay men to participate in preventive HIV vaccine trials; Conf Adv AIDS Vaccine Dev, 212 [poster 92], 1996, Bethesda, MD.

Hays, R., Kegeles, S., & Coates, T. (1990). High HIV risk taking among young gay men. *AIDS, 4*:901-907.

Hays, R., Kegeles, S., & Coates, T. (1996). Unprotected sex & HIV risk taking among young gay men within boyfriend relationships. *AIDS Education & Prevention*.

Higgins, D. L., Galavotti, C., O'Reilly, K. R., Schnell, D. J., Moore, M., Rugg, D. L., & Johnson, R. (1991). Evidence for the effects of HIV antibody counseling and testing on risk behaviors. *Journal of the American Medical Association, 266*(17):2419.

Hoff, C. C., Coates, T. J., Barrett, D. C., Collette, L., & Ekstrand M. (1996). Differences between gay men in primary relationships and single men: Implications for prevention. *AIDS Education and Prevention, 8*(6):546-59.

Hoover, D. R., Muñoz, A., Carey, V., Chmiel, J., Taylor, J., Margolick, J., Kingsley, L., & Vermund, S. H. (1991). Estimating the 1978-1990 and future spread of Human Immunodeficiency Virus Type 1 in subgroups of homosexual men. *American Journal of Epidemiology, 134*:1190-1205.

Hunt, A. J., Davies, P., McManus, T., Weatherburn, P., Hickson, F., Christofis, G., Coxson, A. P. M., & Sutherland, S. (1992). HIV infection in a cohort of homosexual and bisexual men. *British Medical Journal, 305*:561-562.

Hunt, A. J., Weatherburn, P., Hickson, F. C. I., Davis, P. M., McManus, T. J., & Coxson, A. P. M. (1993). Changes in condom use among gay men. *AIDS Care, 5*(4):439-448.

Kelley, J. A., Kalichman, S. C., Kauth, M. R., Kilgore, H. G., Hood, H., Campos, P. E., Rao, S. M., Brasfield, T. L., & St. Lawrence, J. S. (1991). Situational factors associated with AIDS risk behavior lapses and coping strategies used by gay men who successfully avoid lapses. *American Journal of Public Health, 81*(10):1335.

Kippax, S., Noble, J., & Prestage, G. (1997). Sexual safety in the AIDS era: Negotiated safety revisited. *AIDS, 11*:191-197.

Kippax, S., Crawford, J., Davis, M., Rodden, P., & Dowsett, G. (1993). Sustaining

safer sex: A longitudinal study of a sample of homosexual men. *AIDS*, 7:279-282.
Marks, G., Ruiz, M. S., Richardson, J. L., Reed, D., Mason, H. R., Sotelo, M., Turner, P. A. (1994). Anal intercourse and disclosure of HIV infection among seropositive gay and bisexual men. *Journal of the Acquired Immune Deficiency Syndrome*, 7(8):866-9.
Marks, G., Ruiz, M., Richardson, J., Reed, D., Mason, H. R., Sotelo, M., & Turner, P. A. (1994). Anal intercourse and disclosure of HIV infections among seropositive gay & bisexual men. *Journal of the Acquired Immune Deficiency Syndrome*, 7:866-869.
McCusker, J., Stoddard, A., Mayer, K. H., Zapka, J., Morrison, J., & Saltzman, S. P. (1988). Effects of HIV antibody knowledge on subsequent sexual behaviors in a cohort of homosexually active gay men. *American Journal of Public Health*, 78(4):462-467.
McKusick, L., Coates, T., Morin, S., Morin, S. F., Pollack, L., & Hoff, C. (1990). Longitudinal predictors of reductions in unprotected anal intercourse among gay men in San Francisco: The AIDS Behavioral Research Project. *American Journal of Public Health*, 80:978-983.
McLean, J., Boulton, M., Bookes, M., Lakhani, D., Fitzparick, R., Dawson, J., McKechnie, R., & Hart, G. (1990). Regular partners & risky behavior. *AIDS Care*, 6:331-341.
Meyer, I. H. & Dean, L. (1995). Patterns of Sexual Behavior and risk taking among young New York City gay men. *AIDS Education & Prevention*, 7(Supp.):13-23.
Myers, T., Godin, G., Lambert, J., Calzavara, L., & Locker, D. (1996). Sexual risk and HIV test-taking behavior by gay and bisexual men in Canada. *AIDS Care*, 8(3):297-309.
Prieur, A. (1990). Norwegian gay men: Reasons for continued practice of safer sex. *AIDS Education & Prevention*, 2(2):109-115.
Remien, R., Carballo-Dieguez, & Wagner, G. Intimacy & sexual risk behavior in serodiscordant male couples. *AIDS Care*, 7(4):429.
Ridge, D. T., Plummer, D. C., & Minichiello, V. (1994). Young gay men and HIV: Running the risk? *AIDS Care*, 6(4):371-378.
Root-Bernstein, R. (1993). *Rethinking AIDS: The Tragic Cost of Premature Consensus*. New York: Free Press.
Sacco, W. P. & Rickman, R. L. (1996). AIDS-relevant condom use by gay and bisexual men: The role of personal variables and the interpersonal situation. *AIDS Education and Prevention*, 9(5):430-43.
Schechter, M. T., Craib, K. J., Willoughby, B., Douglas, B., McLeod, W. A., Maynard, M., Constance, P., & O'Shaughnessy, M. (1988). Patterns of sexual behavior and condom use in a cohort of homosexual men. *American Journal of Public Health*, 78(12):1535-8.
Schoofs, M. (1997, May). Who's Afraid of Reinfection? *POZ Magazine*, 64.
Service, S. K. & Blower, S. M. (1995, June). HIV Transmission in sexual net-

works: An empirical analysis. *Proceedings of the Royal Society London B Biological Sciences, 260*(1359):237-244.

Snyder, M. & Omoto, A. (1994). Volunteerism and society's response to the HIV epidemic. *Current Directions in Psychological Science, 1*(4):113-116.

Stall, R. D., Ekstrand, M. O., Pollack, L., et al. (1990). Relapse from safer sex: The next challenge for AIDS prevention efforts. *Journal of the Acquired Immune Deficiency Syndrome, 3*:1181-1187.

Stall, R. D., Coates, T. J., & Hoff, C. (1988). Behavioral risk reduction for HIV infection among gay and bisexual men: A review of results. *American Psychologist, 43*(11):878-85.

Tindall, B., Swanson, C., Donovan, B., & Cooper, D. A. (1989). Sexual practices and condom usage in a cohort of homosexual men in relation to human immunodeficiency virus status. *Medical Journal of Australia, 151*(6):318-22.

Torrian, L. & Weisfuse, I. B. (1996). Trends in HIV seroprevalence in men who have sex with men: New York City Department of Health Sexually Transmitted Disease clinics, 1988-93. *AIDS, 10*(2):187-92.

Turner, H. A., Catania, J. A., & Gagnon, J. (1994). The prevalence of informal caregiving to persons with AIDS in the United States: Caregiver characteristics and their implications. *Social Science Medicine, 38*(11):1543-52.

van Griensven, G. J. P., de Vroome, E. M., Tielman, R. A., Goudsmit, J., de Wolf, F., van der Noordaa, J., & Coutinho, R. A. (1989). Effect of human immunodeficiency virus (HIV) antibody knowledge on high-risk sexual behavior with steady and nonsteady sexual partners among homosexual men. *American Journal of Epidemiology, 129*:596-603.

Voigt, R., Scheter, M. T., Craib, K. J., Hogg, R. S., Zadra, J. N., Willoughby, B., Sestak, P., & Montaner, J. S. (1992, July). Increasing condom use but stable numbers of casual and regular partners in a cohort of gay men (1987-91). The Vancouver Lymphadenopathy-AIDS (VLAS) Study Group. *Proceedings of the International Conference on AIDS, 8*:2, C261 (abstract no. PoC 4096).

Winkelstein, W., Jr., Samuel, M., Padian, N. S., Wiley, J. A., Lang, W., Anderson, R. E., & Levy, J. A. (1987). The San Francisco Men's Health Study: III. Reduction in human immunodeficiency virus transmission among homosexual/bisexual men, 1982-86. *American Journal of Public Health, 77*(6):685-689.

Anal Sex and Gay Men:
The Challenge of HIV and Beyond

Onno de Zwart, MA
Marty P. N. van Kerkhof, MA
Theo G. M. Sandfort, PhD

SUMMARY. In this article, the structure and meaning of anal sex among gay men in the era of AIDS are analyzed. Based on sexual script theory and using a grounded theory approach, 71 Dutch gay and bisexual men were interviewed. During each sexual encounter decisions have to be made about whether or not anal sex will take place, who will play what role, and if protection is used. The decisions taken are not only related to individual preferences, but to a large extent also to those of the partner involved. HIV is one, but not the only factor, influencing these decisions. Four distinct scenarios have been identified which structure and give meaning to anal sex: the physical, the intimate, the reciprocal, and the power scenario. Related to these scenarios are obstacles and stimuli to use condoms. In the physical scenario, condoms are an obstacle to bodily pleasure. In the intimate scenario, condoms hinder emotional closeness. In the reciprocal scenario, condoms are disruptive for each act of anal sex. The rules of the power scenario facilitate the integration of condom use. Suggestions are made on how to incorporate these results in HIV prevention. *[Article copies available for a fee from The Haworth Document Delivery Service: 1-800-342-9678. E-mail address: getinfo@haworthpressinc.com]*

Since unprotected anal sex is the main route of HIV transmission for gay men, this behavior has been featured in much of the psychosocial AIDS research during the last sixteen years. This literature is largely focused on the frequency of protected and unprotected anal sex, the partners with whom it takes place, and the influence that personal attitudes toward anal sex might have on individual prevention behavior (see Donovan et al., 1994, for an overview). Rarely have studies examined the motives, decision-making processes, personal strategies, and meanings associated with this sexual act (exceptions include Davies et al., 1993; Henriksson, 1995; Morin, 1981/1986; Odets, 1995; Prieur, 1990; Rofes, 1996). These aspects are, however, of utmost importance if we want to understand anal intercourse in the time of HIV. Without more detailed knowledge about anal sex, researchers and HIV prevention workers will continue failing to comprehend the decisions gay men make about both protected and unprotected anal intercourse.

This article is based on qualitative research carried out in the Netherlands between 1993 and 1995 (Van Kerkhof et al., 1995). Our aim is to examine the structure and meaning of anal sex among gay men in the time of AIDS. In the first part we will discuss the decisions gay men make during anal sex. Specific attention will be paid to two primary issues which face each set of partners: Whether or not anal sex will take place and which role (active or passive) each man will play. In the second part we will assess the various meanings anal sex has for gay men and how these meanings are related to specific obstacles and motivations for using condoms.

An excerpt from the interview with one of our subjects, Casper (age 39 years, all names used are pseudonyms), introduces some of the important qualities of anal sex which we will explore here in more detail. Casper has a steady partner with whom he rarely has anal intercourse as well as another regular sex partner with whom he always fucks.

> When we see each other it always results in that [fucking]; it is our unspoken rule. He likes it when I take him, and I enjoy fucking him. We start sucking each other; after that I begin fingering him till his butt feels really open. Then comes the moment when I tell him that I'm going to take him. A condom is grabbed and he puts it on me. He is very good at doing that. He makes my cock real hard and in a second he has it on me. What I like very much about him–which is one of the reasons why I keep seeing him–is that he is totally into it. That turns me on even more, and so we drive each other totally crazy.

Caspar's account makes clear that several decisions take place during a sexual encounter. These decisions can be analyzed to gain a better understanding of the interaction. Although in this case the sexual act has become a regular routine, decisions have to be made each time about whether or not anal sex will take place, who will play what role, and if protection will be used. This case example also shows the meaning fucking can have for the subject as well as the importance of the interaction with the specific partner.

In reporting our findings we have chosen to use the words of our interviewees, like *fucking*. In our analysis we also frequently use the word *decision* as a way to describe aspects of the sexual interaction; however, the use of this word does not mean we consider sexuality as purely rational. We see sexuality and sexual encounters as a complex and interactive process. In this process, several elements can be distinguished: two (or more) individuals; their interaction; and the physical and psychological context (Davies et al., 1993; Gagnon, 1990).

THEORETICAL CONSIDERATIONS AND METHODS

In our study we used the sexual script theory (Gagnon, 1990; Simon & Gagnon, 1987). A basic assumption of this approach is that people act according to a *script* when having a sexual encounter. These scripts contain the parameters for the sexual interaction, including intra-psychic (motivations, fantasies), interpersonal (interactive cues) and cultural (sub-cultural values placed on anal sex) aspects. Sexual scripts help persons to interpret the sexual situation and to respond to it. Individuals develop their scripts over time based on (sub-)cultural values and personal experiences. In a specific situation two or more gay men encounter each other and define that situation as sexual. On the basis of their scripts, a sexual interaction takes place within that specific physical context. Meanings come about and are the result of these sexual interactions. Scripts help men to make sense of the signals of their partner and to react to these signals.

Procedure. Methodologically, we used the grounded theory approach (Glaser & Strauss, 1967; Strauss & Corbin, 1990). Central to this model is the cyclic nature of the research process: Four rounds of data collection, analysis, and reflection take place. During the first two rounds we interviewed 41 men. On the basis of these interviews we developed concepts to describe the way gay men structure anal sex. In the third phase, 10 men were interviewed. The analysis of these and the earlier interviews made clear that during anal sex, several decisions have to be made. This phase of the study also revealed that various scenarios can be distinguished which structure the sexual encounter as well as give it meaning. In the last cycle we interviewed 20 men, using these interviews to further refine the earlier ideas we had formulated.

The first two authors carried out all interviews, each interview being between ninety minutes and three hours in length. The in-depth, semi-structured instrument focused on concrete descriptions of specific sexual encounters, including where the men had anal sex. All interviews were transcribed.

In recruiting the sample, we sought to identify a diverse group of gay men who would be able to explore the issue of anal sex in detail. To reach potential subjects, we placed ads in a variety of gay magazines and national and local newspapers. We also used the snowball technique. From those who responded we selected 71 men to be interviewed. We ensured diversity in the sample by using key questions with regard to education, age, place of residence, HIV status, experience with specific sexual environments, and relationship status. We included men from the leather community as well as HIV-positive men in the research group so as to examine the special place anal sex may have in the leather scene and the specific experiences of infected men. Further, we interviewed men who had no experience with anal sex so as to analyze their motivation for not engaging in this behavior.

Subjects. We interviewed 71 self-identified gay and bisexual men, all living in the Netherlands. The age ranged from 18 to 63 years, the mean being 36.4, with 37.2% of the sample under 30 years of age. Men differed with regard to their anal sex experience: 30 men had experience with anal sex before the AIDS epidemic started; 31 had their first experiences of anal sex after 1982. Five men had given up anal sex completely, whereas, 5 men had never had anal sex.

Almost a third of the men were from Amsterdam; close to 30% were from one of the other larger cities of the Netherlands; and almost 40% came from other parts of the country. The level of education varied: 14.1% had completed a primary school education, 31% had completed secondary school, and 54.9% had education beyond secondary school.

With regard to relationship status, 29 men (41%) had a steady partner, of whom 9 declared their relationship to be monogamous. The majority of respondents had been tested for HIV: 10% were positive, 43% were negative. Forty-five percent of the sample did not know their serostatus.

The men differed also regarding how important anal sex is to them. For 31 men, anal sex was described as "very important"; 31 men rated anal sex as being "neither important nor unimportant." For 9 men, anal sex was "unimportant." Almost 40% of the men preferred the passive role,

32% preferred the active role, and 20% enjoyed both roles. Most men (73%), however, had experience with both roles. Although the research group cannot be considered a representative sample, it is diverse enough to lend insight into the anal sex experiences of Dutch gay men.

RESULTS AND DISCUSSION

To fuck or not fuck, that is the question. The decision whether to engage in anal sex is an issue in each sexual encounter, regardless if the sex is with a casual contact or with a steady partner. The above example of Casper shows that whether anal sex takes place depends very much on the wishes of the partner. Although Casper likes to fuck, he only rarely has anal sex with his steady partner, because his partner does not like fucking. On the other hand, he almost always fucks with the other partner. Thus, the relative importance which anal sex has for an individual is not necessarily the decisive factor in determining whether fucking will take place. It does, however, influence whether men will take the initiative for anal sex. The more men value anal sex, the more deliberately they will initiate it.

> Being fucked is really a turn on for me, both the experience itself and to fantasize about it. When I meet someone I therefore presume that it will happen. (Kent, 35 years)

For those men for whom fucking is less important, this decision depends more on who their partner is, what his wishes are, and the specific sexual interaction during the encounter.

> It is something on the side. When there is the right mood, I know we will become so intimate that we will go that far. (Joram, 29 years)

During the sexual encounter itself, many factors influence the decision whether anal sex will take place or not. Trust is, for many men, a prerequisite for fucking, although men differ in the kind of trust they desire.

> As the passive partner you open up your ass, that means you trust the other. When there is no trust or when you are made to feel ashamed [for taking the passive role] that can be very humiliating. (Alain, 24 years)

For some men, trust means that they reserve anal sex for their steady partner; others can trust a new partner immediately.

> I will not fuck with a casual contact because then the conditions under which I like it are not met. . . . I reserve fucking for that person with whom I feel really comfortable. (George, 33 years)

> Some you trust right away, whereas others you don't. But those who you don't know that well are often the most exciting. (Ewoud, 26 years)

There are certain factors which can hinder as well as stimulate men to engage in anal sex. For some, physical features of the partner-like the size of his cock-may stimulate them to have anal sex; whereas for others, daunting penis size and other aspects may raise the possibility of pain while being fucked, and therefore, reduce the likelihood of anal sex. For others, emotional factors can also be both an obstacle (e.g., the fear to be penetrated) as well as a stimulus (e.g., love for the partner). Cultural factors also influence the decision. Some men consider anal sex to be unnatural and will therefore not have anal intercourse; whereas, for others, fucking is considered a necessary part of their coming out process.

> Part of my coming out process was fucking, because that's what sex between men is about. At least that was what I thought, and so did all my friends at that time. It had to happen the first time. For me, it was a kind of reward for all my suffering. (Arthur, 24 years)

The fact that sexual encounters are an interactive process means that men will be influenced by different factors with different sexual partners, and by different situations with the same partner.

During the last two decades, AIDS has become an additional factor influencing the decision whether or not to engage in anal sex. For some men in our study, AIDS proved to be a reason for giving up anal sex completely. This was especially true for men who reported anal sex not being important to them and for those who had only practiced it to please their partners (see also Davies et al., 1993). Other men had stopped having anal sex as a result of AIDS for a period of time, but had taken up the practice again in recent years. Apart from a general fear of AIDS, some men had been influenced by the Dutch prevention message which from 1984 to 1992 discouraged gay men to fuck (de Zwart et al., in press).

> They very clearly warned against fucking. And the special gay condoms became available only later. For me, it is like a scale which is in balance again. On the one side there was my wish to be fucked. On the other side was the weight of information against it. And then,

the information became clearer that in certain situations fucking was allowed. (Felix, 38 years)

Many of our respondents had developed their own personal prevention strategies which influence their decision to engage in anal sex or not (see also Gold, 1994; Levine & Siegel, 1992; Mendès-Leite, this volume). Some men fuck only with those men who *appear healthy* or whose serostatus they (presume to) know. Others feel they can fuck with a younger partner but not with men of certain groups. For example, some men do not fuck with Americans. For these men, deciding whether or not to fuck with a particular partner or type of partner has become a part of their risk-management strategy.

Insertive or receptive (active or passive). After the decision is made to engage in anal sex, the next issue to be addressed is which role each partner will take. Most men in our study had a specific role preference. However, as with the decision to have anal sex, what actually happens depends on the interaction during the encounter. The result is that, in spite of their preferences, most men report role-flexibility. For some, that is one of the special things about homosexuality.

> Especially in a longer relationship there has to be dialogue and interplay. That makes homosexuality so special compared to heterosexuality. Everything is interchangeable and convertible. (Edmond, 35 years)

Like the decision to fuck, role-flexibility can depend on a specific partner and can also be influenced by physical aspects. The trust placed in the other is another important factor. For men who prefer the active role, trusting the other is a prerequisite before they let themselves be fucked. These men stress this aspect more than men who normally prefer the passive role. In some cases, one person induces the other quite easily to give up his own preference; whereas on other occasions, men give up their preference more reluctantly. In rare cases, conflicts about role can mean that no anal sex takes place.

> That guy radiated something very submissive, also because he was almost half a head smaller than me. And his submissiveness induced my need to fuck him. Added to that, he kept turning on his back spreading his legs. For me, that was a clear signal that he wanted to be screwed. (Ivo, 30 years)

The frequency of role-flexibility stresses once again the interactive nature of the sexual encounter.

Scenarios. The decision-making process described above is but one element of the experience of anal sex. Based on the transcripts of the interviews, we have distinguished recurrent patterns in the order of behaviors during the sexual encounter. Also, although each encounter has a specific meaning to the participating partners, the different meanings of various encounters can be clustered. These recurrent patterns and clusters of meanings have enabled us to construct the common scenarios which give order and meaning to sexual encounters, thereby helping us to better understand the sexual interactions. Essentially, then, a scenario outlines the action of the encounter, ordering the behaviors and giving them meaning.

In our study we have distinguished four scenarios of anal sex: the physical, the intimate, the reciprocal, and the power scenario. These scenarios are not constants for any given person or couple, but change over time. Each man can also engage in different scenarios with one and the same partner or with different partners. These scenarios seem to be linked to specific obstacles as well as to specific motivators affecting condom use during anal sex. This observation suggests that condom use is part of an interactive, multi-dimensional process and so cannot be reduced to the technical skills of one of the partners (see also Bochow, 1995; Davies et al., 1993; Gold, 1993; Hart & Boulton, 1995; Levine, 1992). We have, therefore, identified the specific motivators and obstacles to the use of condoms for each scenario. We have found that condom use is one factor among others which structures sexual encounters and gives meaning to them.

The physical scenario. The story of Casper at the beginning of this paper is a clear example of anal sex where the fulfillment of bodily pleasures is central to the encounter.

> What I like very much about him–which is one of the reasons why I keep seeing him–is that he is totally into it. That turns me on even more, and so we drive each other totally crazy. . . . I was so horny and he was even working on my nipples, which blew me away. (Casper, 39 years)

In a physical scenario, men start with sexual activities like kissing and sucking, after which one partner fucks the other or gets fucked. The encounter has a physical meaning to the individuals. In this scenario respondents used words like *horniness, good* and *fulfilling* (in a physical sense) to describe their experiences. The significance here lies in the physical pleasure the experience brings to each of the partners individually. A physical scenario can take place with both casual and steady partners. In such situations, condoms can be an obstacle in that they diminish the physical sensations of anal sex. They also disrupt what men describe as the *naturalness* of the interaction; that is, something artificial has to be introduced which interrupts *the flow* of the sex.

> It feels far much better to go bareback into it . . . A condom always fits a bit tight, the heat is different and it [the fucking] is not so smooth. (Ewoud, 26 years)

> They are impractical, no matter what they say–even if it's done in a fun way or even if someone is very good at using them. Putting them on is a technical thing which is not a logical part of the sexual scene. (Olaf, 46 years)

The intimate scenario. The order of behaviors found in this scenario does not differ much from the physical scenario; that is, after activities like kissing and sucking the climax of the encounter is fucking. The meaning anal sex has for the partners is, however, quite different. Anal sex is an emotionally intimate act. It is seen as an expression of closeness and togetherness between the partners.

> At that moment I wanted to get fucked by him. I wanted to feel his dick inside my ass. I was horny for that boy and I loved him so much. I wanted to experience together with him the highest form of intimacy, which is fucking. It gave me the feeling that I was one with him. (Ewoud, 26 years)

In the intimate scenario, anal sex is often considered the pinnacle of a relationship. Most men in our study practiced this scenario in their steady relationships, although for some men casual encounters could have an intimate meaning, as well. The intimacy experienced by the men is expressed in terms of *unity, trust, becoming one,* and *it's so special with him.*

> Fucking is something the two of us share, something we have with no one else. At those moments, you become real close to each other and it really happens that from two persons we become one. Fucking is for us more than a physical feeling; it expresses that we have something special together. (Joram, 29 years)

In intimate scenarios, the problem with condoms is that they hinder the merging with the partner; when condoms are used, the unity is considered to be incomplete.

> The more I care about somebody, the more intimately I feel for him, and the more I see a condom as being an impediment. When I fuck with somebody who is emotionally not that important to me, I focus more on technique and action, and I don't have the feeling that I'm missing anything because of the condom. When, however, I fuck my boyfriend–which happens often–I notice something is missing. Because of that piece of rubber, the direct contact is gone; and what is also very important is that, because of that [the rubber], I can't come in him. (Abel, 26 years)

One of the main functions of condoms–namely, to prevent the giving and receiving of semen–is thus a major obstacle to achieving intimacy (see also Prieur, 1990). Men experience the receiving of semen as a special physical gift of their partner which can symbolize a *super intimacy*. By having their partner's semen in their body, men feel that they carry their partner with them, even when he is gone. Both the men who started fucking before the AIDS epidemic, as well as those whose first experiences were after the advent of HIV, value the meaning of semen in their sexual experiences and fantasies. In terms of exchanging semen, condoms are considered particularly disruptive during sex with steady partners.

> Because you really receive something from someone and you give something of yourself to your partner. The physical feeling of having the semen of someone inside you evokes certain thoughts. Although it may sound weird, it happens that, although my friend has already gone, because of it [his semen inside me] I still remember his presence. (Malcolm, 30 years)

The reciprocal scenario. This scenario differs from the physical and intimate scenarios in its ordering of behaviors. In the reciprocal scenario, both partners fulfill both roles during the intercourse, active and passive, during one sexual encounter. The anal sex can have a physical meaning as well as an intimate meaning, depending on various factors, including the specific partner involved.

> It was quite funny. I said that I wanted to be on top and he replied, 'Me, too.' So, first of all, we had to decide who would go first. We both wanted to give the other the fun of going first, but finally I fucked him. (Malcolm, 30 years)

More respondents who were in a steady relationship practiced this scenario, as compared with men who had only casual partners. Some men preferred this scenario as it stresses *equality* between the partners. In these situations, condoms are seen as an obstacle because of the physical and intimate meanings the fucking may have (as described above). For other men, however, there is the additional problem that the use of condoms disrupt the *natural order* of the sexual encounter twice.

> You are very busy with each other and with the sex and when the time has come you have to get it out of it's wrapping. You really have to do your best to get everything in order again. (Julian, 30 years)

The power scenario. The power scenario differs significantly from the others with respect to both the order and type of sexual activities involved (e.g., bondage, whipping, etc.), as well as with respect to the meaning anal sex has. Central to this scenario is the ritualizing and eroticizing of power and inequality (see also Coxon, 1996). During the encounter, one of the partners has a dominant role, whereas the other partner is submissive. When men in our study described such encounters, the permission of the submissive partner was a prerequisite to engaging in this form of sex.

> The penetration was quick, rough, and wild. I like it most when somebody just gets into you so that you can feel the hard head of his cock inside something soft. You feel the friction inside and the pushing against the prostate. (Joost, 22 years)

> Penetration is really something which is part of an S/M scene. You feel that the submissive is totally surrendering himself. Certainly, when he is tied up, he is totally defenseless. At that moment I am the one who decides what is going to happen. That gives me a great feeling. I don't let up then, because if I did, I wouldn't have any more control, and as a top, I can't let that happen. (Manfred, 35 years)

Condoms are reportedly used more often in power scenarios than in other situations. Our results contrast with other studies which have analyzed power in sex between men. For example, Davies and Weatherburn (1991, p. 122) have concluded that when "desire is articulated through a rehearsal of domination rather than a celebration of equality" more unprotected sex occurs.

In our opinion there are some reasons why power scenarios lend themselves more to condom use than do other forms of interaction. First of all, the power scenario is more often carried out with casual partners with whom sex in general is more protected (Bochow et al., 1994; McLean et al., 1994). Power scenarios are also characterized by set rules, including the permission of the submissive person, as already mentioned. It seems that to add an extra rule, such as using condoms, poses no particular problem, as it is only one rule of many. Finally, during power scenarios, sex paraphernalia are often used (e.g., toys, clothing, etc.), making it easier to accept condoms as simply another object to be incorporated in the play.

> Although I couldn't see it, I knew he had put on a condom. When the head of a cock is coming into your hole, you feel the rubber around it. We have, however, strict arrangements about that and we trust each other. (Joost, 22 years)

More research is needed to establish whether more protected sex takes place in the context of power scenarios and what mechanisms are in place which induce men to use condoms in these situations. Such research seems particularly relevant at a time when S/M and other power-related sexual activity is becoming more popular (Tatchell, 1994; Coxon, 1996).

CONCLUSION

Anal sex is a complex, dynamic process during which gay men make several decisions. An interactional perspective regarding sex between gay men, taking into account the context and meaning sexuality has, is a prerequisite for coming to understand such a process. In this paper we have shown that gay men consider various factors, including the reactions and preferences of their partners and the specifics of the situation, when deciding whether or not to fuck and what role to play. The influence of the partner in a sexual encounter is thus of utmost importance.

Scenarios can be described as a means of analyzing how sexual behaviors are ordered during an encounter and as a way of identifying the meanings anal sex may have. AIDS is only one factor among others which influences the decisions made during anal sex. There is also a variety of obstacles and motivators regarding condom use which are related to the scenarios themselves. We have also demonstrated that anal sex can have various meanings, depending on the sexual situation, including: the deepest expression of intimacy; the pinnacle of a relationship; the fulfillment of bodily pleasure; the celebration of equality; and the ritualization of power differences. When condoms hinder experiencing such meanings, it is logical that gay men would decide not always to use them.

Our results are based on the experiences of Dutch gay and bisexual men. Other recent studies in the United Kingdom and Australia have also indicated the importance of the meaning of anal sex (Bartos et al., 1996; Flowers et al., 1996).

If HIV prevention wants to address the real needs of gay men it has to begin by valuing the different emotional and symbolic meanings anal sex has. In developing HIV prevention activities, it is important to take into account the specific obstacles to condom use which are related to specific scenarios. This means prevention activities have to acknowledge the tensions which can exist between the wish to experience intimacy, the desire to receive semen, and the desire for physical pleasure vs. the need to use condoms. HIV prevention activities face the challenge of starting a real dialogue with gay men about their experiences with anal sex, about the meaning it has for them, and about the personal prevention strategies which they have developed. Such dialogues, whether they take place in face-to-face interactions, group discussions, or media debates, offer a chance to bring together the lived experience of gay men and the insights of AIDS research and prevention.

BIBLIOGRAPHY

Bartos, M. R., Middleton, H. & Smith, G. (1996). Gay men in regular relationships and HIV risk. *XI International Conference on AIDS*, Vancouver, Poster TuD2698.

Bochow, M. (1995). Datenwüsten und Deutungsarmut. Zu Defiziten in der präventionsorientierten AIDS-Forschung am Beispiel der Zielgruppe homosexuelle Männer. *Zeitschrift für Sexualforschung 8*(1):39-48.

Bochow, M., Chiarotti, F., Davies, P., Dubois-Arber, F., Dür, W., Fouchard, J., Gruet, F., McManus, T., Markert, S., Sandfort, T., Sasse, H., Schiltz, M., Tielman, R. & Wasserfallen, F. (1994). Sexual behaviour of gay and bisexual men in eight European countries. *AIDS Care, 6*(5):533-549.

Coxon, A. P. M. (1996). *Between the Sheets. Sexual Diaries and Gay Men's Sex in the Era of AIDS*. London: Cassell.

Davies, P. M. & Weatherburn, P. (1991). Towards a general model of sexual negotiation. In: P. Aggleton, P. Davies, & G. Hart (Eds.), *AIDS: Responses, Intervention and Care*. London: Falmer Press, 111-125.

Davies, P. M., Hickson, F. C. I., Weatherburn, P. & Hunt, A. J. (1993). *Sex, Gay Men and AIDS*. London: Falmer Press.

de Zwart, O., Sandfort, Th. G. M. & van Kerkhof, M. P. N. (in press). No anal sex please: We are Dutch. A dilemma in HIV prevention directed at gay men. In: Th. G. M. Sandfort (Ed.), *Social Policy, Research and Prevention Responses to HIV/AIDS. The Case of the Netherlands*. London: Taylor & Francis.

Donovan, C., Mearns, C., McEwan, R. & Sudgen, N. (1994). A review of the HIV-related behaviour of gay men and men who have sex with men. *AIDS Care, 6*(5):605-617.

Flowers, P., Sheeran, P., Smith, J. A. & Beail, N. (1996). Combining quantitative and qualitative methods to understand unsafe sex among gay men. *XI International Conference on AIDS*, Vancouver, Poster MoD1862.

Gagnon, J. (1990). The explicit and implicit use of scripting perspective in sex research. *Annual Review of Sex Research*, 1:1-43.

Gold, R. (1993). On the need to mind the gap: On-line versus off-line cognitions underlying sexual risk taking. In: D. J. Terry, C. Gallois, & M. McCamish (Eds.), *The Theory of Reasoned Action: Its Application to AIDS Preventive Behaviour*. Oxford: Pergamon, 227-252.

Glaser, B. & Strauss, A. (1967). *The Discovery of Grounded Theory*. Chicago: Aldine.

Hart, G. & Boulton, M. (1995). Sexual behaviour in gay men: Towards a sociology of risk. In: P. Aggleton, P. Davies, & G. Hart, *Safety, Sexuality and Risk*. London: Falmer Press, 55-67.

Henriksson, B. (1995). Risk factor love: The symbolic meaning of sexuality and HIV prevention. *Proceedings of AIDS in Europe–The Behavioural Aspect. Berlin, edition sigma*, 2:115-133.

Hoccquenghem, G. (1978). *Homsexual Desire*. London: Allison & Busby.

Levine, M. (1992). The implications of social constructionist theory for social research on the AIDS epidemic among gay men. In: G. Herdt, & S. Lindenbaum, *The Times of AIDS: Social Analysis, Theory and Method*. Newbury Park: Sage Publications.

Levine, M. & Siegel, M. (1992). Unprotected sex: Understanding gay men's participation. In: J. Huber, & B. Schneider (Eds.), *The Social Context of AIDS*. Newbury Park: Sage Publications.

McLean, J., Boulton, M., Brookes, M., Lakhani, D., Fitzpatrick, R., Dawson, J., McKechnie, R. & Hart, G. (1994). Regular partners and risky behaviour: Why do gay men have unprotected intercourse? *AIDS Care*, 6(3):331-341.

Morin, J. (1981/1986). *Anal Pleasure & Health: A Guide for Men and Women*. Burlingame: Yes Press.

Odets, W. (1995). *In the shadow of the epidemic. Being HIV-negative in the age of AIDS*. Durham: Duke University Press.

Prieur, A. (1990). Gay men: Reasons for continued practice of unsafe sex. *AIDS Education and Prevention*, 2(2):110-117.

Rofes, E. (1996). *Reviving the Tribe: Regenerating Gay Men's Sexuality and Culture in the Ongoing Epidemic*. New York: Harrington Park Press.

Simon, W. & Gagnon, J. (1987). A sexual scripts approach. In: J. H. Geer & W. T. O'Donohue (Eds.), *Theories of Human Sexuality*. New York: Plenum Press, 363-383.

Strauss, A. & Corbin, J. (1990). *Basics of Qualitative Research: Grounded Theory, Procedure and Tactics*. London: Sage Publications.

Tatchell, P. (1994). *Safer Sexy. The Guide to Gay Sex Safely*. London: Freedom Editions.

van Kerkhof, M. P. N., de Zwart, O. & Sandfort, T. G. M. (1995). *Van achteren bezien. Anale seks in het aidstijdperk*. Amsterdam: Schorer.

Imaginary Protections Against AIDS

Rommel Mendès-Leite, PhD

SUMMARY. In this article, we analyze the psychosocial mechanisms for managing the risk of HIV infection; we call these imaginary and symbolic protections. Their definition is simple and based on the observation that being aware of prevention guidelines does not necessarily lead people to adopt long-term and systematic behavioral changes. Instead, people use psychosocial processes that will give them the impression that they are taking no risks. We show how these processes are intrinsically related to the symbolic management and manipulation of the relationships to others, thus demonstrating that certain forms of risk-taking are non-rational. *[Article copies available for a fee from The Haworth Document Delivery Service: 1-800-342-9678. E-mail address: getinfo@haworthpressinc.com]*

Unsafe sex is not irrational, but a different sort of rationality. (Davies et al., 1993, p. 53)

In the beginning of the AIDS epidemic, the prevention discourse was largely based on the rather simplistic assumption that publicizing safer sex guidelines was enough for people to apply these guidelines effectively and *rationally*. (For a summary and review of prevention approaches see Davies et al., 1993.) Since that time, research has shown that avoiding HIV infection is at odds with individualistic, rationalistic and functionalist models of risk management which are based on controlling one's own behavior. These models are ineffective when it comes to managing both one's own and one's partners' behavior, and when the issue is to protect oneself by involving the other (Paicheler, 1992).

The complexity of the factors involved in the sexual risk-management of HIV infection has been identified in several studies. These works are generally focused on the role of different behaviors and sexual practices in the context of various situations and interpersonal interactions (Bochow, 1993, 1995; Davies et al., 1993) as well as on the importance of social support (Prieur, 1990) or on the role of unconscious motivations (Odets, 1992). Among European researchers, there is virtual unanimous agreement that unsafe sexual practices are not necessarily caused by irrational behavior, but rather by a different form of rationality (Davies et al., 1993; Mendès-Leite, 1992).

Data collected in France and Brazil (1990-1994) from homosexually-identified subjects and other men who have sex with men, using methods derived from social anthropology and qualitative sociology, illustrate the type of thinking which is operative. Based on 120 face-to-face interviews and field observations, we noted the existence of a phenomenon which we called *imaginary protections* (Mendès-Leite, 1992; Mendès-Leite & de Busscher, 1992) (see Table 1). Our work reveals that most individuals acknowledge the necessity of using various prevention techniques to avoid HIV-infection. Yet people sometimes apply the official prevention guidelines by giving them a different meaning.

This process of reassigning meaning involves a kind of symbolic *manipulation* of preventive techniques, which allows these practices to be drawn closer to the person's own cognitive framework. The person is then able to perform particular sexual behaviors while assuming he is taking no risk. Such is the case, for instance, for the subject who, instead of systematically using condoms during anal intercourse, only does so based on his sex partners' appearance and lifestyle (what McKusick et al. (1985) call *selective strategies*). While, epidemiologically, such a strategy may seem irrational due to its ineffectiveness, it is nevertheless quite logical from the perspective of the person involved. In his own way, he is striving to attain a primary goal of prevention–namely, to avoid having unprotected sexual contacts with an infected person. He does so by subjectively defining who those infected people are.

The individual's subjective transformation of prevention guidelines can have three main functions: first, to transpose the categories of official prevention messages into the sociocultural and conceptual framework particular to the individual as social actor (*transference*); second, to simplify or alleviate constraints while providing the impression that the chosen behavior is still effective (*simplification*); and third, to dialectically negoti-

TABLE 1. Forms of Imaginary Protection

A. Identification Devices

Game of appearances	Selection of partners based on their appearances (physical size, hygiene, feel, etc.)
High-risk areas	Selection of partners based on their social and/or geographical origins
Age of danger	Selection of partners based on generational criteria
Sexual identity	Selection of partners based on their sexual identity (heterosexual, homosexual, or bisexual)
"Seedy looks"	Selection of partners based on their known or inferred socio-sexual lifestyles (in/out of the gay scene, promiscuous, etc.)
High risk practices	Selection of partners based on their known or inferred sexual practices (anal intercourse, sadomasochism, etc.)

B. Maintenance Devices

Unspoken agreement	One or both partners in a relationship is in denial about having multiple partners: "Let's not talk about it and it won't exist."
Serial monogamy	A series of monogamous or "faithful" relationships with different people
Relationship built on trust	To grant one's unknown partners minimal trust, and maximal trust to familiar partners
Blood oath	Reassurance based on feeling (friendship, passion, love)

C. Exorcism of the Disease

Exorcism through screening	Belief in an innate or acquired immunity due to repeated testing with negative results
Exorcism through having a condom available	Acquired confidence based solely on having a condom in one's pocket or wallet
Exorcism through reducing the number of partners	Trust in a strategy based on reducing the number of partners or on one form of fidelity considered as sufficient

ate a re-adaptation between one's own sexuality and the social standards dictated by prevention (*negotiation*). In addition, *imaginary protections* are structured according to two basic factors, i.e., the relationship to the *Other* and the contrary (or paradoxical) effects of prevention messages themselves.

THE PHENOMENON OF IMAGINARY PROTECTIONS

> Risk is not a material thing; it is a very artificial intellectual construct which lends itself particularly well to social assessments of probabilities and values. (Douglas, p. 56)

Anthropology has demonstrated the existence of a *prevention concept* in all cultures and social systems (Dozon, 1992). One universal feature is the attempt to preserve social interactions by representing proactive control over events (Héritier-Auger, 1991). As a cultural construct, prevention and prevention-related behaviors "can only be studied in reference to all the representations people have of the disease, the body, hardship, and the world" (Fainzang, 1992, p. 19). In the context of sexually transmitted diseases, the representations of the *social imagery of sexualities* (sex, gender, sexual categories and orientations, lifestyles and sexual lifestyles, etc.) are very important. Individuals will interpret prevention guidelines according to their sociocultural backgrounds, giving these guidelines a meaning which will make their implementation possible. This perfectly rational mechanism does not deny the significance of a prospective attitude toward protecting oneself from disease. On the contrary, individuals will appropriate protective behaviors and give them meaning precisely because they value them. The contents of the resultant protective measures and attitudes may, however, appear to others to be contradictory. Anthropological research conducted in Africa provides examples of many such social behaviors related to prevention which would not–in strict epidemiological terms–be considered "rational" (see Augé, 1984; Fainzang, 1989, 1992).

Looking at *imaginary protection mechanisms* for HIV from an anthropological perspective offers interesting clues regarding various aspects of this phenomenon. Obviously, from a conceptual point of view, the categories used by epidemiology as well as those embraced by anthropology or qualitative sociology are not necessarily in agreement, since these disciplines are not based on the same type of logic (Coppel, Boullenger & Bouhnik, 1993). Here we are interested in the socio-anthropological study of the interaction between common knowledge and public health categories. Analysis has shown, as Ferrarotti (1983, p. 51) points out, that "far from merely reflecting the social context, the individual appropriates, adapts, filters, and re-translates this context, while projecting it into another dimension, which is ultimately that of his or her own subjectivity. He or she cannot disregard the messages of prevention, but he or she also does not take them in passively; he or she re-invents the messages moment by moment." The prevention discourse in France concerning homosexually-identified men and other men who have sex with men has been trying for some time to reflect the diversity of people's lifestyles. Yet, with the exception of information concerning sadomasochism and other hard-core sexual practices, all material distributed to this target group describes sexual acts as being interchangeable (de Busscher, 1995), without taking into account the diverse meanings various sexual practices may have due to the individual's social, sexual, emotional, and lifestyle context. That is, higher risk acts, such as unprotected anal intercourse, are depicted as being easily replaced by lower risk acts, such as using dildos.

METHODS

Both sociological and anthropological methods were used in the collection of data for this research, including field ethnographic observations and life stories which were compiled using an interview grid and a semi-structured questionnaire. Data thus collected were placed in their sociocultural context, using both subjective indicators as provided by interviewees and quantitative information collected by the researchers.

The sample was composed of males with homosexual experience, with no restriction as to age or sociosexual characteristics, including sexual identity. Field research was conducted in two countries, France and Brazil. In each country, subjects were recruited from three different environments: (a) a major city with its suburbs (Paris and Rio de Janeiro); (b) large or middle-sized cities (Nantes, France and Fortaleza, Brazil); and (c) a rural area with relatively small urban centers (the Vendée province and the Deux-Sèvres district for France; the hinterland in the Ceara State in Brazil).

The so-called "snowball" method was used for subject recruitment. As for the French part of the research, 57 interviews were conducted with an average duration of two hours each (sometimes extending to four or even six hours). In Brazil, 41 interviews were conducted, based on the same grid as in France and with a similar duration. In addition, a further 22 interviews with people identifying themselves as "gay" were included. Lastly, survey material obtained during the research was also used in order to refine the analysis of social representations of sexuality and related practices and behaviors.

Using the Alceste software, taped and transcribed interviews from both samples were submitted to a vocabulary analysis based on context and on a descending, hierarchical classification. They were also grouped by primary themes. This software considers the discourse on a given subject matter as a consistent corpus and, from there, divides the text into equal-sized segments. It then identifies the occurrence rate for words, word pairs and sentence segments within the whole corpus in order to check how vocabulary units (at least the most frequent ones) are combined. This procedure identifies if word X is mostly used with word Y, whereas, word Z may be most commonly associated with word W. Therefore, an area A can be identified that includes several segments of the text where words X and Y are often combined, whatever their actual locations in the corpus, and an area B, where words Z and W are frequently found. Finally, the role of chance in the occurrence of the word associations can be tested using the Chi-Square method.

This form of analysis allows us to understand structurally how ideas or concepts consciously or unconsciously lead from one to the other, without employing any particular psychological theory of word association. It also allows us to conduct a systematic search on the vocabulary and thus places us at the heart of social actors' representations of sociosexual categories and identities.

Based on the resultant separation of words into text segments, according to their associations, we can then conduct a detailed analysis of the vocabulary found in each of the different classes that have been established using the descending, hierarchical analysis in order to reconstruct the representation structure which underlies social actors' discourses on a particular subject matter.

RESULTS

Social categories which, on the surface, may seem obvious are not always unequivocal. For instance, such a concept as *faithfulness* may involve nuances, sometimes subtle, which do not necessarily identify it with monogamy. Someone may clearly discriminate between physical and emotional faithfulness, the latter being considered as more significant–and not necessarily tied to–an exclusive, sexual partnership:

> It's the heart, I think. Staying true to a feeling of love for someone. I mentioned earlier that I had had relationships with other men during those five years, but I don't feel like I was unfaithful, because I didn't love them. I did not give myself to them, really. But, a few years ago, when I gave myself fully to the man whom I'm still with, I gave him something more than just my body. I gave him my every thought, I gave him this rare feeling–too rare maybe–which is the feeling of love that is deep within oneself. I did not give this to the other men I met–I just gave them my body for a little while. (VDS, 28 years, sales clerk)[1]

> Faithfulness is psychological; it is not a physical thing. (PAR, 70 years, architect)

Many (homosexual as well as heterosexual) couples thus admit to an "extramarital" sex life, which does not necessarily jeopardize their primary relationship.

> I'm very jealous, so faithfulness is pretty important to me. But the way I see it, as I meet more and more guys, faithfulness is something almost impossible for gay people. Actually, I never came across a one-hundred-percent faithful male relationship. When and if relationships work, it's because each partner has sex on the side every now and then, and they come back together in the evenings. (VDS, 25 years, programmer analyst)

> For me, fidelity is not something sexual. I think I'm faithful to Paul in my own way. Granted, I have sex on the side, but mostly these things are not very important or not important at all. (PAR, 37 years, computer console operator)

Even when fidelity is associated with monogamy, its duration may be too limited to really guarantee security, giving way to short-term, serial monogamy.

Other questions are raised by cultural variables such as the *unspoken agreement*, a form of denial used to keep up the appearance of sexual and affective fidelity, using a highly traditional pattern found in many societies.

> No, it's just the way it was, but we were officially faithful to each other. We didn't talk about it because I knew he knew and he knew I knew. Why ruin the relationship we had, which was rare and precious? Just because of a few quickies? (PAR, 38 years, pop singer)

> I think that it's not having sex outside of a relationship that prevents things from working out. [. . .] Yes, I think that you can be faithful without necessarily being exclusive. [. . .] Ah yes, what I wanted to say is that I don't believe in automatically being completely open about it with your partner when you are attracted–or sexually attracted–to someone else. You may decide to be completely sincere and reject hypocrisy and tell your partner everything–the smallest attraction such and such person may induce. But you still end up hurting your partner! I think you destroy what you have, you can destroy the other person. (VDS, 32 years, biologist)

Categories related to sex and gender may also have an influence, albeit in a more limited number of cases. For example, the clients of transvestite prostitutes interviewed by Mendès-Lopes who, because they are not "exactly" homosexuals, do not consider unprotected anal intercourse as unsafe.

Socially stigmatized sexual practices are sometimes branded as being the source of evil to be avoided. Young heterosexual North-Africans living in the Paris suburbs, studied by Boullenger, reported "that you could catch it [HIV] only through butt-fucking" (Coppel, Boullenger & Bouhnik, 1989, p. 48). By the same token, women in charge of the regional branch of a major French AIDS service organization thought that their non-governmental organization (NGO) was not *ethically allowed* to bring up safer sex issues with young people because these women considered sexual practices other than vaginal penetration as abnormal. For these women, safer sex had nothing to do with using condoms, although they spoke unreservedly in support of their use. Safer sex had to do with "abnormal" acts (e.g., sex without penetration). Therefore, because condoms refer to vaginal penetration, that is, a *normal* practice, it did not need to be raised (see also, Spencer, 1993).

As previously stated, *imaginary protection* strategies do not imply that the individuals affected do not know about or do not believe in the effectiveness of HIV prevention. On the contrary, faced with the social demand to rationalize (sexual) behaviors and practices perceived by most as belonging to a natural or even instinctive framework, people create cultural responses which allow for both the preferred sexual practice and protection against HIV. One possible response is to use a specific rationality which seems equivalent to, or even *more logical* than officially promoted risk management strategies.

Many authors working in the fields of sociology and risk anthropology agree that the individual's assessment of his or her situation derives from his or her specific practices. As reminded by Duclos (p. 41) "it is a 'limited' rationality which makes possible dealing with immediate concerns while 'forgetting' larger questions which one is incapable of grasping." Even though this observation was made about certain types of prevention which are completely different from the ones researched here, it applies to HIV sexual transmission risks, as well. While being aware of the lethal risk of AIDS, people have a differential management of prevention techniques. In addition to the primary objective of protecting themselves from being infected, they *naturally* add the goal of lessening the restrictions called for by HIV prevention.

Difficulties concerning prevention practices vary, and different individuals with different sociocultural backgrounds perceive them differently and organize them in distinct hierarchies. For some men, the main stumbling block is the feeling of latex against the skin; for others, it may be the abrupt discontinuity involved in actually putting on a condom. Some other people have no problem using condoms for anal (or vaginal) intercourse, but are incapable of doing so for fellatio. Still others have difficulty refraining from anal intercourse or in reducing the number of partners. All of these people are thus led to make pragmatic choices and to favor the prevention techniques that are most feasible for them.

These limitations to prevention have already been taken into account in several countries where the "safe sex" target (maximum protection from HIV during all sexual acts) was rejected in favor of the more realistic "safer sex" approach (de Busscher, 1995). In Western Europe, for example–albeit with differences among countries–the official prevention discourse abandoned the notions of curtailing the practice of anal intercourse or promoting condom use for fellatio.[2] Several surveys have demonstrated that maximum risk reduction is not achievable for many men who have sex with men (Bochow, 1995; Davies et al., 1993; Mendès-Leite, 1993a). French prevention strategies targeted at these men, however, include a growing number of recommendations aimed at reducing the number of partners or extolling fidelity and monogamy. A leaflet which was reprinted this year specifically added such advice to its existing contents. Although this type of campaign may appear to be outdated in the English-speaking world, in France, sex *with everybody and anybody* is strongly discouraged and cruising *anywhere and everywhere* is looked down on. This type of campaign reinforces people's adopting attitudes related to imaginary protection, such as selecting their partners based on their appearances, lifestyles, and geographical origins:

> Since the AIDS epidemic started, my sex life has changed in the sense that, when I have an afternoon encounter, I try to assess whom I'm dealing with. I want to know whether he is likely to . . . to be contaminated. I don't know, from his looks, I guess. If I can see it? Well, I don't know–there are those people that you see only once, but whom you trust more than others, as opposed to someone you meet every day in a cruising area. This type of person I wouldn't go with, because it's too much, that would be tempting the devil. [. . .] But let's say that if someone looks healthy–although it doesn't mean much . . . I don't know, but someone who looks healthy, who is well-dressed and everything, I would probably trust him more, even though it would be wrong. I know it would be wrong because, after all, I would know nothing about him. (NAN, 36 years, bus driver)

> The AIDS issue doesn't bother me so much since we're in Niort. If I were in Paris, obviously it would mean either wearing a rubber or having no sex. Whether I like condoms or not, I would have used them, I think. (VDS, 26 years, special education teacher)

> I know guys who died from AIDS. Yes, several guys, but it wasn't in Niort. These were people who . . . who traveled a lot. (VDS, 74 years, retired)

> I had it [anal intercourse] only once, I'd say. And it was in Paris with a Parisian–well, with someone living in Paris. But when I've had relationships here, as far as I know, it [the issue of anal intercourse] was never brought up except maybe with one person once, but that's almost never. It only happened to me in Paris. I think that this type of sex is not as common in the Provinces. Yes, that's what I think. [. . .] So it's probably meaningful that . . . I've had the opportunity to talk about this during my short trips to Paris and to either do it or turn it down whereas here, in this region, I never had to resist in the least. [. . .] I have wondered whether there is some kind of self-censorship in the Provinces–or at least here–or some kind of fashion trend, an imitation of standardized, Parisian gay sexual practices. I have no ready-made answer to this, but I think it's a little of both. (VDS, 32 years, biologist)

This way of thinking is similar to that of men who assume that they may stop regularly using condoms because they have decreased the number of their partners (for a discussion of this issue, see Mendès-Leite, 1993a).

To continue having a large number of sexual partners–but only with carefully selected men–is an example of having adapted a preferred sexual lifestyle through a subjective re-interpretation of prevention guidelines. This kind of adaptation has also been identified among young suburban heterosexuals in France, albeit with certain unique features (Coppel, Boullenger & Bouhnik, 1989), and among divorced/separated people (Bastard & Cardia-Veneche, 1992).

As stated above, individuals try to view their sexual preferences according to a prevention logic and adapt this logic to their likings and proclivities. Another example is how people take advantage of the fact that the discourse regarding the use of condoms for fellatio is very ambiguous, so they create messages to favor their own preferences.

> No, I don't use condoms for fellatio, only for anal intercourse. It was never demonstrated that fellatio was unsafe. It may involve some

risk factors, but since it's very limited compared to . . . Well, I think the odds are much lower, so . . . (VDS, 25 years, programmer analyst)

I don't like anal intercourse, either with or without a condom. That way, I eliminate an awful lot of risk. Now, as for fellatio, when the other guy doesn't come in your mouth . . . But I'm still careful. I've had sex with guys whom I knew were HIV-positive because they told me so or I had heard about it. In these instances I didn't kiss as much. I would be very careful to not let my partner come in my mouth. You can feel when the guy is about to come. Once, a guy was holding my head, but normally I can feel it. I can always feel when the other guy is reaching climax. (PAR, 22 years, student)

I'm unsure about fellatio. The medical community is completely divided on this issue. Some doctors say that it can be transmitted this way while others deny it. [. . .] I hate tasting plastic when I go down on someone. It's very unpleasant. How do I decide to wear a condom or not? It all depends on my partner–if he wants me to, I wear a condom, no big deal; if he doesn't want me to, then I generally don't feel like wearing one since doctors' opinions are highly divergent on this issue. What I am most careful about is to avoid getting cum in my mouth. It means that, whenever my partner looks like he's reaching climax through fellatio, I will try to prevent him from coming directly in my mouth, but it wouldn't bother me at all. (PAR, 21 years, student)

It's obvious that, whenever penetration occurs, a condom is involved. But there's the issue of fellatio. I, for one, can't suck on plastic, I just can't. It involves a risk, even if it is minimal, but I know there's a risk. Nobody ever came in my mouth. I try not to suck for too long. [. . .] Yes, I receive blow jobs as well. Do I wear a condom in this case? Well, no, I don't. (PAR, 37 years, computer console operator)

There's still much more uncertainty about fellatio than about anal intercourse. I was told that the risk was minimal. Let's say I believed it. And fellatio is a very common practice among gays–you do it all the time. I don't always get cum in my mouth, but still. I could easily withdraw but I think that keeping it in my mouth and then spitting it out is enough. I wash afterwards and my partners do, too. (PAR, 23 years, student)

Similarly, one man we interviewed presented himself as "completely and only active," but admitted during the interview to having been the receptive partner during sexual intercourse with men whom, given their physical appearance, he deemed to be "safe."[3]

Another variation is finding new *tools* for safer sex to replace those officially recommended, due to products being too expensive or unavailable where sex is taking place. These new *tools* are used in the belief that they are equally effective. For example, people may use oil-based (Vaseline, Nivea cream, or butter) instead of water-based lubricants. Boullenger provides a more dramatic example: a young suburban Parisian did not want to miss an orgy and, since he did not have a condom, he substituted a plastic shopping bag (Coppel, Boullenger & Bouhnik, 1993).

Finally, repeatedly receiving a negative result on the HIV test sometimes has the symbolic value of an *exorcism of the disease*. When testing is done on a regular basis, it is perceived to be a vaccine of sorts.

> I get screened every third month. (PAR, 26 years, wine waiter)

> Yes, about twice a year. Each negative test takes the doubt away. Sometimes I feel like I'm lucky, that's true. Yes, I think that it's a healthy practice; one should get tested twice a year. (PAR, 37 years, computer console operator)

> I get tested on a quarterly basis. I'm negative, I don't have AIDS. I don't have cancer either although I smoke four packs a day. [. . .] I love blow jobs, and I know why I love them so much. It is because of this feeling I have of complete dominance over my partner. I just love it, makes me crazy. Do I swallow the cum? Yes, it happens, depending who I'm with. No, I'm not scared about it, not at all. I tell them right away that I blow without condoms because if they tell me they want to wear one, I tell them to forget about the whole thing. [. . .] Guys come in my mouth, yes. Of the hundred men or so who have been in my mouth, there certainly were a few who were positive. Oh yes, I'm completely aware of this. If it bothers me? No, not at all. [. . .] I get screened every three months, give or take a month. What surprises me is that I'm still negative; I get a kick out of it. (PAR, 38 years, pop singer)

> I get tested twice a year and my last test was two months ago. The reason I do it is because you don't know how this disease evolves. You may get infected and only come down with it ten years afterwards. And I don't remember what I was doing ten years ago . . . Of

course I know what happened then, but I wasn't paying attention. That's why you have to get tested twice a year. It makes sense to me. (PAR, 34 years, manager in the fashion industry)

My lover and I get screened regularly three to four times a year. [...] Well, because even if you're careful, since both of us have sex on the side, we want to get screened as a precaution. Obviously, if we were completely faithful to each other from a sexual point of view, we wouldn't need to. But since we sometimes have affairs, it's like staying on the safe side, and getting screened is a far more honest attitude towards the people you meet. (NAN, 36 years, bus driver)

Repeatedly receiving a negative HIV result may be interpreted in terms of innate or acquired immunity to possible infection through unprotected anal intercourse or to repeated unsafe intercourse with HIV positive partners. As suggested by de Busscher, this may bear reference to a rather free interpretation of the Pasteurian vaccination principle, i.e., being in contact with an inactive or weak strain of a virus may result in developing antibodies for this specific virus and becoming immune to its effects (de Busscher, personal communication).

Like testing, condoms may also have a symbolic value which reduces their efficacy, for example, when people use them infrequently or when they have condoms in their pockets or wallets (like a lucky charm) but do not use them. This leads us to an observation similar to that of Zonabend (1989) about the *trust* atomic plant workers place in gauges for radioactivity measurement. She noted that "there is a symbolic and metaphoric transformation of these objects [...]. From this perspective, there is little need to question their reliability, since it is all a matter of belief" (*ibid.*, p. 51). The circumstantial use of the various forms of fidelity or reducing the number of sexual partners according to the various *selective strategies* are further "metaphorical transformations" (Zonabend, 1989) of prevention guidelines which may have ambiguous consequences, to say the least.

These *symbolic manipulations* (with their very concrete ramifications) do not invalidate the goal of prevention, but they do bring to light some of the limitations of prevention work and its inherent dilemmas. There are limits to a *social contract* between two partners in which they promise to take on a shared responsibility in terms of AIDS prevention. As hypothesized by Dozon (1992, p. 33), this does not mean "that [this contract] cannot actually be an incentive for using prevention techniques, but rather that it is bound to identify how complicated and diverse prevention strategies are and their association with various configurations of meaning which, through often paradoxical tricks, are adapted to the 'relational' contents."

IMAGINARY PROTECTIONS AND "THE OTHER"

La prévention n'est jamais sans risques. [Prevention is never without risk.] (Kipman, 1994, p. 17)

The relationship to others is one basic problem of HIV prevention because the practices being addressed are symbolically significant. To protect oneself against AIDS and other STDs involves a dual management: managing oneself and managing relationships with others, which inherently implies being cautious of others. If one is to control one's acts in order to avoid a sexually transmitted disease, infection can only happen through another person. Therefore, the *Other* directly or indirectly represents *danger*. When the prevention discourse tells us to avoid unprotected intercourse or to limit the number of partners, we are warned against none but the *Other*. In contrast, when official messages proclaim that one has to be faithful to his companion or that he may have unprotected intercourse provided that he is both certain of himself *and* of his only (or regular) partner being HIV negative, the prevention discourse then teaches that one may trust only certain *Others*.

The main *imaginary protections* we identified in our interviewees' responses which have to do with the image of the *Other* we called *identification devices* and *maintenance devices* (see Table 1).

By adapting terms used by Fainzang (1989), we identify two different types of *Others* in this rationale: the *Familiar Other* and the *Unknown Other*. Relationships with these two are not the same, and neither is the level of trust. Yet the difference between these two categories is not fixed; on the contrary, it is fairly dynamic, and a partner easily goes from being one to the other. This is particularly true in the case of someone getting to know a partner and therefore gaining his (previously undeserved) trust. This difference can be trivial in social relationships, but this dynamic may be the cause of manipulations in meaning which become *imaginary protections*.

At first, one finds out whether the *Unknown Other* is actually a *Dangerous Other* (borrowing terms from Clatts & Mutchler, 1989) through his appearance (*game of appearances*), his social or geographical origin (*high-risk areas*), the generation he belongs to (*age of danger*), his lifestyle (*seedy looks*) or his sexual preferences (*high-risk practices*). If the person does not bring "*reassurance*, one can reject him or choose to have sexual intercourse without penetration (or sometimes fellatio) or intercourse with condoms. An alternative is that the possible partner, who matches the selection criteria established by the individual, is considered a *Safer Unknown Other* with whom he can avoid taking all or some of the usually recommended precautions right away or just for a limited period of time. Later on, including this partner in the *safer* category can be reinforced and knowledge of him will turn him into a *Familiar Other* (*relationship based on trust*). Acquired trust and sometimes feelings like friendship or love emerge and will then play a crucial role (*blood oath*). Once the partner is considered a *Safe Familiar Other*, various mechanisms can enter into play so that he avoids becoming a *Dangerous Other*. Strategies connected to fidelity and found in the category *maintenance devices* (*unspoken agreement, serial monogamy*) are very important in this respect (see Table 2).

CONCLUSION

One of the benefits of the imaginary protection theory is that it can be generalized to populations other than men who have sex with men. Our suggested approach makes it possible to understand not only what representations are implemented in HIV risk management, but also what types of sexual imagery are operative, and how personal prevention strategies interract with ideological constructs (e.g., prevention as defined and presented by public health authorities; de Busscher, 1995). Imaginary protection theory also can reveal how prevention and related representations function for social actors and how these representations determine real-life behaviors.

As we have seen, the representations described by imaginary protection allow for a rational risk management of sexual HIV transmission, although it is a rationality which is radically based on peoples' daily experience. During each new sexual encounter, partners act based on thought and action patterns which are developed in individual life stories, and these individual life stories are in turn part of collective stories. Partners enact their social and cultural experiences and develop a subjective perception of the actual risk-taking, dialectically using the objective information they have about the disease.

Imaginary protection theory therefore makes it possible to account for issues which are at the interface of theoretical knowledge and practical experience (Bourdieu, 1980) as these protections establish a link between the development of representations for *Others* and for HIV at individual, group, and societal levels.

As we can see, the boundary between symbolic and actual experience is very permeable and the obstacles to prevention are therefore many and of

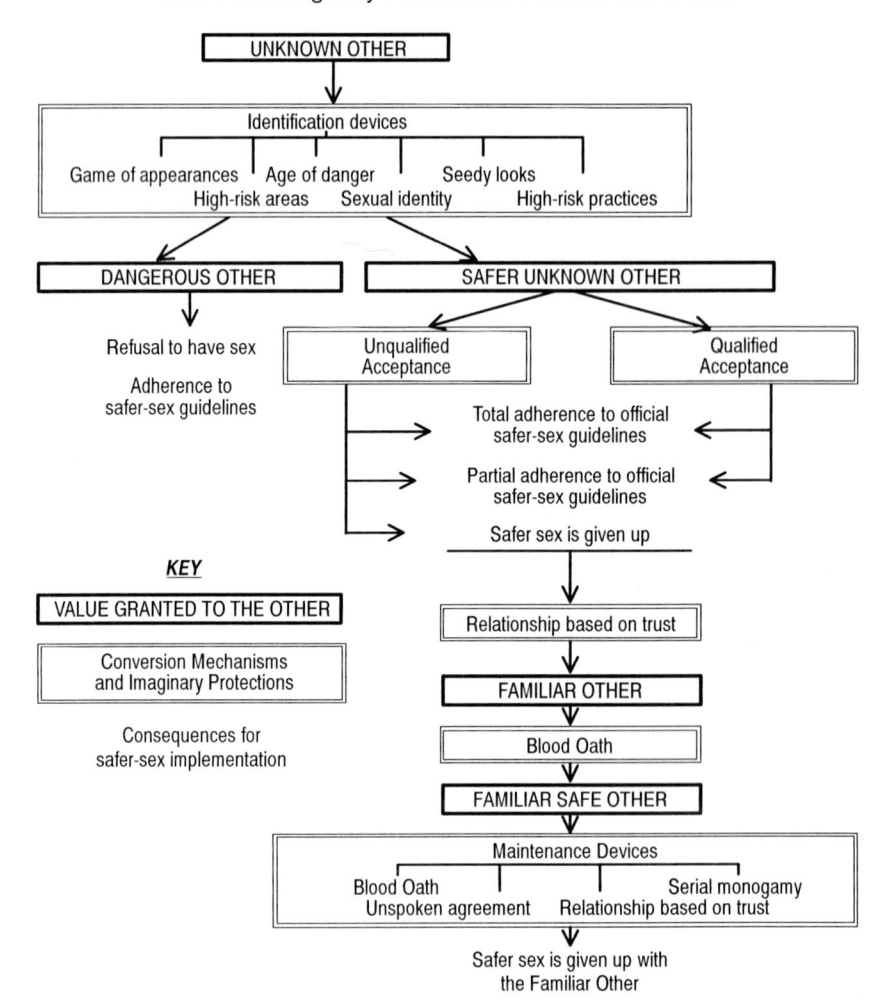

TABLE 2. Imaginary Protections Conversion Process

```
                         UNKNOWN OTHER
                              │
                              ▼
        ┌─────────────────────────────────────────────┐
        │            Identification devices           │
        │  Game of appearances   Age of danger   Seedy looks  │
        │     High-risk areas   Sexual identity  High-risk practices │
        └─────────────────────────────────────────────┘
              │                              │
              ▼                              ▼
    ┌──────────────────┐          ┌──────────────────────┐
    │ DANGEROUS OTHER  │          │  SAFER UNKNOWN OTHER │
    └──────────────────┘          └──────────────────────┘
              │                       │              │
              ▼                       ▼              ▼
    Refusal to have sex      ┌─────────────┐  ┌─────────────┐
                             │ Unqualified │  │  Qualified  │
    Adherence to             │ Acceptance  │  │ Acceptance  │
    safer-sex guidelines     └─────────────┘  └─────────────┘
                                  │                  │
                         →  Total adherence to official  ←
                            safer-sex guidelines
                         →  Partial adherence to official ←
                            safer-sex guidelines
                         →  Safer sex is given up
                                       │
                                       ▼
                          Relationship based on trust
                                       │
                                       ▼
                                FAMILIAR OTHER
                                       │
                                       ▼
                                  Blood Oath
                                       │
                                       ▼
                             FAMILIAR SAFE OTHER
                                       │
                                       ▼
        ┌─────────────────────────────────────────────┐
        │             Maintenance Devices             │
        │  Blood Oath                   Serial monogamy │
        │  Unspoken agreement    Relationship based on trust │
        └─────────────────────────────────────────────┘
                                       │
                                       ▼
                          Safer sex is given up with
                              the Familiar Other
```

KEY

- VALUE GRANTED TO THE OTHER
- Conversion Mechanisms and Imaginary Protections
- Consequences for safer-sex implementation

a very diverse nature, their connections to actual sexual practices being complex. It is only by acquiring detailed descriptions from individuals–not only regarding their concrete sexual practices, but also about their sexual imagery and their concepts of sexuality–that we can take into account the many variables which impact on the diverse (homo)sexualities which exist. In doing so, we have the foundation for developing more adequate prevention policies and campaigns.

NOTES

1. The region where each interviewee was living is indicated (PAR for Paris and suburbs; NAN for Nantes and suburbs; and VDS for Vendée-Deux-Sèvres), as well as age and occupation. These data were collected August 1990–April 1992.
2. The Dutch prevention policy is an example of a shift from maximum protection to achievable risk reduction. Instead of recommending that homosexuals use condoms for anal intercourse, early campaigns urged men to stop practicing anal sex altogether. This message has since been abandoned (Duyvendak & Koopans, 1991).
3. For example, he said he avoided having sexual intercourse with "skinny people," whom he perceived as being "questionable, from a health point of view." This seems to relate to the mass media publishing photographs of emaciated terminally-ill AIDS patients, as well as to traditional views on underweight people (concerning this latter point, see Fischler, 1987).

BIBLIOGRAPHY

Aiach, P. (1994). La prévention: Une idéologie de progrès? *Agora (30), Idéologies de la prévention.*
Augé, M. (1991). Ordre biologique, ordre social: La maladie forme élémentaire de l'événement. In M. Augé & C. Herzlich, (orgs.), *Le Sens du Mal. Anthropologie, Histoire, Sociologie de la Maladie*, Paris: Editions des Archives Contemporaines.
Bastard, B. and Cardia-Voneche, L. (1992). Les choix et les comportements affectifs et sexuels face au sida. Une étude sociologique auprès de personnes séparées ou divorcées. *Rapport de recherche à l'ANRS, Centre de sociologie des organisations.*
Bochow, M. (1993). Les déterminants des comportements à risques. In R. Mendès-Leite, (org.), *Sociétés (39), Sexualités et Sida*. Paris: Dunod.
Bochow, M. (1995). La sexualité à risque existe-t-elle? In R. Mendès-Leite, (org.), *Un sujet inclassable? Approches sociologiques, littéraires et juridques des homosexualités.* Lille: Cahiers GKC.
Boullenger, N. (1993). Réseau de sociabilité et pratiques sexuelles dans un site de banlieue parisienne. In A. Coppel, N. Boullenger & P. Bouhnik, *Les réseaux d'échange sexuels et de circulation de l'information en matière de sexualité chez les jeunes des quartiers à risque.* Paris: GRASS, IRESCO, ANRS.
Calvex, M. (1992). La sélection culturelle des risques du sida. *Final ANRS Research Report.* Rennes: Institut Régional du Travail Social de Bretagne.
Coppel, A., Boullenger, N. & Bouhnik, P. (1993). *Les réseaux d'échange sexuels et de circulation de l'information en matière de sexualité chez les jeunes des quartiers à risque.* Paris: GRASS, IRESCO, ANRS.
Davies, P., Hickson, F., Weatherburn, P. & Hunt, A. (1993). *Sex, Gay Men and AIDS.* London: The Falmer Press.

de Busscher, P.-O. (1996). Non-profit organization "Santé et Plaisir Gai" and safer sex development in France (1988-1994). In ANRS (dir.), *Les homosexuals face au sida. Rationalités et gestion des risques*. Paris: ANRS.

de Busscher, P.-O. (1994b, September). The development of safer-sex as an ideology. France, 1989-1994. In Friedrich, D. & Heckmann, W. (eds.), *AIDS in Europe–The behavioral aspect: Framework of Behavior Modifications*. Berlin: Sigman.

Douglas, M. (undated). Les études de perception du risque: Un état de l'art. In J.-L. Fabiani & J. Theys, (orgs.), *La société vulnérable. Évaluer et maîtriser les risques*. Paris: Presses de l'École Normale Supérieure.

Douglas, M. & Wildavsky, A. (1982). *Risk and Culture. An Essay on the Selection of Technological and Environmental Dangers*. Berkeley: University of California Press.

Dozon, J.-P. (1992). Limites d'une organisation "rationnelle" de la prévention. In N. Bon, P. Aiach & J.-P. Deschamps, (orgs.), *Comportements et Santé. Questions pour la prévention*. Nancy: Presses Universitaires de Nancy.

Duclos, D. (undated). La construction sociale des risques majeurs. In J.-L. Fabiani & J. Theys, (orgs.), *La société vulnérable. Evaluer et maîtriser les risques*. Paris: Presses de l'École Normale Supérieure.

Duyvendak, J.-W. & Koopmans, R. (1991). Résister au Sida: Destin et influence du mouvement homosexuel. In M. Pollak, R. Mendès-Leite & J. Van Dem Borghe, *Homosexualités et Sida*. Lille: Cahiers GKC.

Fainzang, S. (1989). *Pour une Anthropologie de la maladie en France. Un regard africaniste*. Paris: Éditions de l'École des Hautes Etudes en Sciences Sociales. (Cahiers de l'Homme, Nouvelle Série XXIX).

Fainzang, S. (1992). Réflexions anthropologiques sur la notion de prévention. In N. Bon, P. Aiach & J.-P. Deschamps (orgs.), *Comportements et Santé. Questions pour la prévention*. Nancy: Presses Universitaires de Nancy.

Ferrarotti, F. (1981). *Histoire et histoires de vie. La méthode biographique dans les sciences sociales*. Paris: Librairie des Méridiens.

Fischhoff, B. (undated). Gérer la perception du risque. In J.-L. Fabiani & J. Theys (orgs.), *La société vulnérable. Evaluer et maîtriser les risques*. Paris: Presses de l'École Normale Supérieure.

Heritier-Auge, F. (1991). Inceste. In P. Bonte & M. Izard, *Dictionaire de l'Ethnologie et de l'Anthropologie*. Paris: PUF.

Kipman, S. (1994). Prudence et prévention. *La revue Agora. Idéologies de la prévention* (30).

Liandre, H. (1994). Les homosexuels et le "safer sex." Contribution psychanalytique à la prévention du sida. *Final Research Report to ANRS Laboratoire de Psychologie Clinique, Université de Paris VII*.

Lys, M. (1994). La prévention, une folie. *La revue Agora, Idéologies de la prévention* (30).

Macintosh, M. (1968). The homosexual role. In K. Plummer (ed.), *The Making of the Modern Homosexual*. London: Hutchinson.

Maneu, E. (1994). La prévention entre responsabilité et coercition. *La revue Agora. Idéologies de la prévention (30)*.

Mendès-Leite, R. (1988). Les apparences en jeu. *Sociétés (17)*. *Entre hommes, entre femmes*. Paris: Masson.

Mendès-Leite, R. (1991). La culture des sexualités à l'époque du sida: Représentations, comportements et pratiques (homo)sexuelles–une recherche qualitative dans les départements des Deux-Sèvres et de la Vendée. In M. Pollak, R. Mendès-Leite, R. & J. Van Dem Borghe, *Homosexualités et Sida*. Lille: Cahiers GKC.

Mendès-Leite, R. (1992). Pratiques à risque: Les fictions dangereuses. *Le Journal du Sida* (42). Paris: Arcat Sida.

Mendès-Leite, R. (1993a). Sur quelques protections imaginaires de contagion par voie sexuelle. *Hommes entre eux (Saintes, juin 1992)*: *Première rencontre des acteurs de prévention. Entre gens (2)*. Vanves: Agence Française de Lutte contre le Sida.

Mendès-Leite, R. (1993b). A Game of Appearances. The 'Ambigusexuality' in Brazilian Culture of Sexuality. *Journal of Homosexuality* (25, 3). New York: The Haworth Press, Inc.

Mendès-Leite, R. (1994). "Comment" ou "combien"? Multipartenariat sexuel et gestion des risques du sida. *Quel Corps?* (47-48), *Sexualités imaginaires–Imaginaires sexuels*.

Mendès-Leite, R. & de Busscher, P.-O. (1992). Les représentations et les vécus homos et bisexuels à l'époque du sida: Les départements de la Vendée et des Deux-Sèvres, Partial Report to AFLS and non-profit organisation Gay'titudes, Paris, Groupe de Recherches et d'Études sur l'Homosocialité et les Sexualités. (Abridged version published in R. Mendès-Leite, (1994)). *Un sujet inclassable? Perspectives sociologiques, juridiques et littéraires des homosexualités*. Lille: Cahiers GKC.

Mendès-Leite, R. & de Busscher, P.-O. (1993). La gestion d'une épidémie au long terme. *Sida: Le combat. Les lettres françaises* (hors série). Paris.

Mendès-Leite, R. & Mendès-Lopes, N. (1994, Septembre). Cahier Ethnographique. Presentation to the annual meeting of the research team *La construction sociale des sexualités en Europe du Sud*, Paris.

Mendès-Lopes, N. (1994). "The tranvestite, the woman and the client: A socio-anthropological approach of transvestite prostitution." Presentation to the "Sex industry" session of the *AIDS in Europe–The Behavioural Aspect international conference*, Berlin, September.

McKusick, L. et al. (1985). AIDS and sexual behavior reported by gay men in San Francisco. *American Journal of Public Health* (75, 5).

Mutchler, K. & Clatts, M. (1989). AIDS and the dangerous other: Metaphors of sex and deviance in the representation of disease. *Medical Anthropology* (10).

Odets, W. (1992). Unconscious motivations for the practice of unsafe sex among gay men in the United States, Poster presented at the VIIIth International AIDS Conference, Amsterdam (PoD 5191).

Oliviero, P. (1992). Sida et représentations sociales des liquides du corps. Final report for research funded by Ministère de la Recherche et de la Technologie, Paris, LPSARLC/EHESS, ANRS.

Paicheler, G. (1992). Connaissances, représentations sociales et comportements: Les logiques préventives. In N. Bon, P. Aiach & J.-P. Deschamps (orgs.), *Comportements et Santé. Questions pour la prévention.* Nancy: Presses Universitaires de Nancy.

Prieur, A. (1990). "Gay men: Reasons for Continued Practice of Unsafe Sex," *AIDS Education and Prevention* (2,2).

Spencer, B. (1993). Le *safer sex* et les rapports dits "sans pénétration": Est-ce bien normal? In R. Mendès-Leite (org.), *Sociétés (39) Sexualités et sida.* Paris: Dunod.

Vollaire, C. (1994). Contre une vision paranoïaque de la prévention: La communauté comme lieu de l'equivocité. *La revue Agora* (30), *Idéologies de la prévention.*

Zonabend, F. (1989). *La presqu'île au nucléaire.* Paris: Éditions Odile Jacob.

Desire, Cultural Dissonance, and Incentives for Remaining HIV-Negative

Wayne Blankenship, MA

SUMMARY. This article, written from the personal observations of an HIV prevention coordinator in San Francisco, discusses some of the current challenges for gay and bisexual men's primary HIV prevention efforts. Psychological issues of personal motivation and identity formation are looked at within the framework of gay culture, pop culture, and the larger heterosexual culture emphasizing their influence on the lives of HIV negative men. The article also looks at age-specific dimensions, comparing the needs of adult men with those of much younger gay and bisexual men. Renewed energy and fresh ideas will be called for to make HIV prevention interventions relevant to the lives of these men. Though the examples and qualitative data cited are from San Francisco, similar phenomena are noted from other cities with gay networks within the U.S. and internationally, suggesting that the experience of San Francisco men will be relevant to prevention providers in any other locales. *[Article copies available for a fee from The Haworth Document Delivery Service: 1-800-342-9678. E-mail address: getinfo@haworthpressinc.com]*

I was surprised to hear what I thought to be a very California new age risk reduction strategy from a European visiting San Francisco recently. He explained that, though he didn't use condoms for anal sex, he believed he would remain HIV negative because of his positive attitude about life. Apparently, personal rationalizations around sexual risk are worldwide phenomena. Conflicting messages regarding sex and risk also seem inherent in many cultures, within gay subcultures and even within our own *culture* of HIV prevention work.

Traditional HIV prevention strategies assume that the way in which we make decisions around sex, often in the middle of the night, are basically identical to the decisions we make during the day at work. I am interested in discussing the possibility that these may be very different, depending on the notions about sex, desire, and risk we have created as a result of cultural messages. In this respect, much could be learned about the influences of culture by comparing the successes and problems faced by different countries regarding sexual risk. What are we to learn from the differences in continued HIV risk among men who have sex with men in various industrialized countries? How do we explain these differences: Climate? . . . Public policy? . . . The inhibiting effects of organized religion?

In this article, I would like to share some thoughts on the current challenges facing HIV prevention efforts in the US, drawing on my personal experience as a coordinator of HIV prevention services for adult gay/bisexual men in San Francisco, observations of gay male pop culture in the 1990s, and data from a qualitative research project in which I was involved. (All quotes from study subjects are taken from transcripts of 1 1/2 to 2 hour interviews of adult gay or bisexual San Francisco men. This study was not designed as a cross-section of men in this city, but was over-sampled for African-American men, Latino men, and men with a history of recreational drug use, not including alcohol or sex for drug exchange).

CULTURAL DEFINITIONS OF SEX AND DESIRE

In qualitative interviews in San Francisco (San Francisco AIDS Foundation, 1997), we discovered that men who engage in unprotected sex can express elaborate personal rationalizations or cultural folk beliefs around the concept of risk. Often fragile, these explanations are nonetheless useful to an individual in explaining: *I, an HIV negative man, seem to have some natural immunity to HIV (or if I have sex with a person I trust, I have reduced my risk)*.

Fragile, seemingly illogical assumptions often exist around topics which are themselves shrouded in mystery, or around subjects rich in conflicting cultural messages. Cultural messages about sexuality in the U.S. certainly fit this scenario. Many men learn that sexual desire is a powerful force; that we do not have to control our desires because desire controls us. Good sex, for males, is often defined as out-of-control sex, something simultaneously sublime and dirty, existing on some other plane of experience. I often sense that we don't want to know too much about it, as if unraveling its mysteries would take away its power.

An advertising poster for a gay erotic video titled *Bad Moon Rising* reads, "These hunters knew only one law: The Law of the Flesh." Apparently, traditional laws are not really applicable in this arena of male sexuality. Desire, if it's really strong, can outweigh the laws of logic. This belief can easily be used to rationalize away the moralistic, be-a-nice-boy, have-safe-sex message which characterizes many under-funded, over-simplified, inoffensive, censored campaigns produced by well-intentioned AIDS service organizations. It should not come as a surprise that some individuals who initially changed behaviors out of compliance to a temporary crisis are now bored with safe sex. For them, the stereotypical idea that gay men were irresponsible beasts before the epidemic but are now ultra-responsible and safe may have recently backfired. The dissonance between the law of the land and the law of the flesh may have disturbing long-term consequences.

SYMBOLIC MEANINGS OF SAFER SEX

Many men in our current research group reiterate the decrease in physical sensation and loss of erections which are associated with condom use. A few men describe in great detail that the introduction of condoms in a sexual situation carries for them all the negative associations of loss, pathology, etc., which have resulted from fifteen years of the epidemic. One man explained that a condom reverses the mood of sex from a pleasurable to a displeasurable, even depressing one. As time progresses, it's not unlikely that these kinds of negative symbolic meanings may become stronger and more prevalent in disproportionately-affected groups of men. Will our HIV prevention efforts be able to address these issues and provide the skills training/psychological support to overcome them?

Not surprisingly, some have perceived our prevention mission as an anti-sex movement. We are accused of being, judging from our funding sources, in bed with big government. A popular music lyric I've heard in gay dance clubs and sex clubs proclaims, "People are still having sex. This AIDS thing's not working." I could easily spend years pondering the implications of such a statement, but suffice it to say, traditional approaches are correctly perceived as biased and sex-phobic. And so the stage is set for widespread distrust of the messenger and the message. After all, as men, we know that sex is not about logic, anyway. It's about desire, risk, guts, rebellion, luck, fate . . . is it not?

> I think there's a kind of selfishness that comes along with that business of fucking somebody. They just feel like I'm a man, I wanna do this the way I want to and if I'm feeling passionate and I want to fuck you without a condom, that's what's gonna happen. (Latino male respondent)

I would assert that a new focus for gay men's prevention might be male sexual patterns of risk in general, since many attitudes and assumptions held by gay men may more likely be the result of growing up male than of growing up gay. This may help explain many of the conflicting desires faced by adult gay men in cities with large gay populations. Here, anonymous or recreational sex may seem institutionalized in gay networks, while skills related to dating, intimacy and relationship-building may appear more difficult to learn and may appear to be unsupported by the sexual culture of the city.

THE DESIRE TO FIT IN (SOMEWHERE)

Some young men understandably may confuse AIDS identity with gay identity. Men, especially in AIDS epicenters, may mistake seroconverting as being their rite of passage into the gay community. A new goal for HIV/STD prevention should be to make sure that other rites of passage are in place. All humans share a desire to fit in somewhere, perhaps none more so than those of us who are different from the rest, those of us who have waited so long to find our place in the world. A 26-year-old in our study described his feelings as a teenager:

> I thought, just being gay, I was already HIV positive. . . . In school, that's like, in *Newsweek,* like hearing it in class and stuff . . . all you knew was that gay people were dying, and it was a gay disease, and I figured that since I liked men, and I knew I did, that I would–that that's how I was going to die.

Another study participant, 27 years of age, said, "When I was younger, I didn't have very many limits. I think I wanted to sort of seroconvert. It sort of, uh, gave a definition."

Especially for those who are particularly concerned about acceptance by the larger heterosexual culture–but who have not personally witnessed the effects of the disease–seroconverting may be seen unconsciously as one of the few options for any type of acceptance and social services. I will never forget the words of a man with AIDS I knew ten years ago, "It's funny, but it will be a lot easier to tell my parents that I have AIDS than that I'm gay." This is why our mission must include confronting institutionalized homophobia and heterosexism as barriers of prevention.

Recent data from studies investigating younger men document rates of unsafe sex and seroconversion sometimes twice that of older men (San Francisco Department of Public Health, 1992; Stall, 1992). The media, and even some researchers, mischaracterize this data to mean that younger men have stopped having safe sex. (This interpretation fits nicely with the only media sound bite about prevention for the last decade: Studies show gay men still having unsafe sex.) However, the younger men in question had never received the targeted education their older counterparts had supposedly discarded, and therefore they hadn't changed their behavior at all. I am confident in saying that younger men, throughout twelve years of public schooling, have not received one message or skills training about developing a healthy sexuality as a gay or bisexual man. Yet many prevention programs assume that they come to us as self-assured adults, skilled in negotiating safety in any sexual situation.

Some men, young and old, who move to San Francisco looking for acceptance, find that as in every culture, some are more accepted than others. Increasing one's threshold of risk to fit into a relationship or peer group is not unique to gay men, though their risks–precisely because they are sexual risks–may seem to be unnecessary and foolish in the face of a life-threatening disease. This desire to fit in, to find a group of peers despite the presence of risk, does not mean that these men are maladjusted, suicidal or psychologically crippled. I am critical of prevention pundits like Walt Odets (1995) for overgeneralizing from clients in therapy to all gay men, pathologizing our lives further by characterizing us all as sad victims of survivor's guilt and post-traumatic stress disorder. HIV prevention efforts often add to this victim mentality by not seeking new and healthy models: by relying on the language of addiction and recovery to talk about sexuality (for example, relapse and prevention case management); and by limiting our dialogue to identifying problem individuals and intervening in their lives for their own good. One survey subject noted: "You can't drag every person out there who's going to put themselves at risk into therapy."

Some strong psychological data dispute the victim role of gay men. One study concluded from a sample of 208 men that, while there was evidence of increased substance abuse disorders and depressive (situational) disorders, there was no correlation for syndromal depression when compared to other populations (Williams et al., 1991). The challenges of the past two decades may have actually accelerated the psychological development of a great many gay men. I suspect that a simple need for belonging and a confusion of gay identity with HIV-positive identity fuels new seroconversions for some. And until recently, I've believed this problem to be a San Francisco phenomenon. But researchers elsewhere are hearing similar rationales–in Paris, for example, where seroconversion is also merging with gay identity, reasons for risk-taking being described, as in this article, in terms of "a psychological rationalization distinct from logic" (Lisandres, 1994). The implication is clear: all cities with gay male networks, not just AIDS epicenters, may eventually be faced with a similar challenge.

RISK AS A POSITIVE CONCEPT

Men learn early in life: Nothing ventured, nothing gained. Risk is an essential component of success. For most gay or bisexual men, risk-taking was necessary in constructing a positive sexual identity. Rather than expecting us to eliminate risk, we should be asking the questions: Given personal values around sexual behaviors, what's an acceptable level of risk for you? What risks do you want to avoid or at least decrease in frequency? Despite the tendency within prevention work to go for absolute safety, we may be able to accept a much more complex range of risk than campaigns now portray.

The Swiss psychologist Hans-Peter von Aarburg has raised some very challenging ideas for us to consider: risk as a way of breaking through unbearable social restraints; risk as a way of challenging fate; risk as a necessary part of individual growth. Such positive concepts of risk must be added to the landscape of prevention practice (von Aarburg, 1996).

Just as defining ourselves as cheerful condom distributors would not be an acceptable role in 1998, oversimplifying a topic as complex as gay male sexuality to only a few slogans and truisms is unacceptable, as well, now over fifteen years into the epidemic. One prevention worker we recently interviewed criticized HIV prevention efforts for restricting our discussion to only simplistic ideas:

> They [gay men] don't have any reason to trust us. . . . We have never said listen, we know what it's like for you to be in a bookstore, late at night, wanting some action, and feeling disgusted when you leave. We know what it's like for you to have sex in the park. . . . We've never validated those things because we powder-puff them for the government.

REMAINING NEGATIVE FOREVER AND OTHER RADICAL ACTS

In San Francisco, the gay press has suggested a split they label as *viral apartheid* to describe the differing agendas of HIV-positive and HIV-negative men. Primary and secondary prevention services for these two groups are often discussed as either/or propositions, and HIV negative men have felt as timid about taking services away from positive men as providers have felt in even using the politically-loaded words *uninfected* or *HIV-negative*. The atmosphere is heavy with distrust, blame, and as always, underfunding.

Images of successful, older HIV-negative men are still rare in the mainstream media and even in the gay press (the latter usually reflecting either a cult of youth and a body fascism, as described by some of the men we interviewed, or an overwhelming preoccupation with HIV). It might be observed that one of the ironic effects of AIDS has been the killing of the notion that gay men can be happy, successful, sexy older adults.

A 1995 newspaper insert entitled *Good Dog*, designed by the San Francisco AIDS Foundation and San Francisco Department of Public Health, proposed the community discussion: What Do HIV Negative Men Say They Want Out of Life? and went on to give these responses: A good dog. A nice apartment. True love. A life that doesn't always revolve around HIV. Resources listed on the reverse side pointed men to every social, sports, and spiritual group in town other than HIV services. Certainly, the specific needs of HIV negative men have changed over time. We assumed that primary prevention was always directed toward HIV negative men. How is it that they perceive we haven't addressed them?

And how should secondary prevention be approached? Should we stress protecting HIV negative partners or HIV positive individuals' protecting themselves from reinfection or other STDs? Ironically, our earlier HIV primary prevention message of assuming every partner is positive has backfired in this large (50%) current population of positive men in San Francisco. Some tell us they still play by our rule. One man reported that "I assume everyone is positive," consequently assuming there's no need for safer sex.

POSSIBLE DIRECTIONS

The application of new harm reduction strategies to our task suggests that we should consider adopting a new concept of sexual enhancement, within a new field of health promotion. I find a good example in the work of San Francisco physician, Dr. Lisa Capeldini, who talks about the health benefits of sexual activity: great cardiopulmonary workout, increased limb flexibility, and stress reduction.

Even the conservative family magazine, *Reader's Digest*, ran an article explaining that sex boosts the immune system. Why do we seem to be so far behind in advocating for the benefits of lower risk sexual activities and the advantages of a larger, rather than a limited, sexual repertoire? Perhaps it's time to create a team of publicly-identified HIV-positive men–a '90s version of the Rubbermen–to serve as hands-on safe sex facilitators in public sex environments, thereby proving confidence in our message that (even HIV positive) men can have rewarding sex without transmitting the virus. Bold new approaches which provoke community discussion, renew energy around the topic, and validate the altruistic behavior of gay men as volunteers, caregivers, and sexual partners throughout the epidemic, need to be explored.

We must begin to unravel the links between drug use and sexual decision-making. Instead of naively proclaiming that drugs and alcohol lead to increased unsafe sex, we have to face the reality that for some, drugs serve as a coping mechanism to reduce stress. For others, who are scarred by homophobia, sex phobia, or physical abuse, self-medication with drugs may be the only way they presently allow themselves to experience sex at all. For men in recovery from addiction, reincorporating a concept of healthy sober sex is of primary concern; HIV prevention aftercare programs are needed as continuations of existing recovery programs.

San Francisco has identified mini-epidemics of HIV which demand specially designed programs: young gay men as a subset of gay/bisexual men; methamphetamine (speed) users (Lewis & Ross, 1995); men of color who don't identify with the white gay community; men experiencing grief over the loss of loved ones; HIV negative men in relationships interested in the skills of negotiated safety (unprotected sex between seronegatives); and men in serious life transitions (career changes, relocations, relationship changes, etc.). Rather than spending energy identifying risky *individuals* and *groups,* we could better focus on *life circumstances* which would tend to increase risk-taking for most normal, well-adjusted individuals.

A new intensive weekend retreat called Boy Meets Boy has been developed in Los Angeles by the Gay and Lesbian Community Services Center to create the time and space for new discussions about sex, intimacy, and relationships. A few Stop AIDS groups in Northern Europe have offered similar retreats for several years–with government funding.

Bolder approaches need to take on policy makers around issues which affect HIV prevention and sexual health. Many adult gay men have learned the skills to successfully advocate for changing the system. These skills need to be applied to new targets, for example, the educational system, which currently can't protect sexual minority students from harassment and violence, much less educate about sexuality and risk. But we can't take on the system alone. New allies are needed, since public education seems now in the hands of parents and religious leaders who disregard sound prevention science. The most striking example of cultural contradictions in HIV prevention is found in the fact that, in the U.S.A., condom manufacturers are still prevented from advertising on commercial television stations. Prevention advocacy must be invented in areas, like this one, where it does not yet exist.

A brochure from Seattle, Washington titled Welcome to Gay City reads, "No more memorial services. No more AIDS protest. No more AIDS fundraisers and NO MORE fucking red ribbons. Imagine gay men counting gray hairs, not T-cells. Imagine no more new HIV infections." Only very recently have we discussed the importance of validating gay men's lives and our contribution to the world as productive adults. If I don't value my life, I'm certainly not going to take steps to protect it. The need for role models of successful, sexy, happy, over-forty gay men is obvious. The epidemic should compel us to use what we know to confront the effects of heterosexism, and to push our allies (researchers, policy makers) to do so, as well. Until providers begin to address the cultural contradictions about sex, monogamy, intimacy, and personal risk, we will continue to implement short-sighted, socially-acceptable interventions, rather than long-term, culturally-appropriate prevention programs.

REFERENCES

Communication Technologies. (1990). A report on HIV-related knowledge attitudes and behaviors among Minneapolis/St. Paul gay/bisexual men: Results from the first population-based survey. Unpublished report prepared for the Minnesota Department of Health.
Lewis, L. & Ross, M. (1995). *A Select Body*. London: Cassell.
Lisandres, H. (1994). Les Homosexuels et le Safer Sex: Contribution Psychanalytique a la Prévention du SIDA. *Recherche à l'ANRS*.
McKusick, L., Coates, T., Morin, S. F., Pollack, L., & Hoff, C. (1990). Longitudinal predictors of reductions in unprotected anal intercourse among gay men in San Francisco: The AIDS Behavioral Research Project. *American Journal of Public Health*, 80(8):978-983.
Odets, W. (1995). *In the Shadow of the Epidemic*. Durham: Duke University Press.
San Francisco AIDS Foundation and the Center for AIDS Prevention Studies.

(1997, March). A qualitative interview study of 92 gay and bisexual males regarding the risk of HIV and sexual behavior. Report of Findings.

San Francisco Department of Public Health AIDS Office. (1992). San Francisco Young Men's Health Study. San Francisco: Department of Public Health.

Stall, R., Barret, D., Bye, L., Catania, J., Frutchey, C., Henne, J., Lemp, G., & Paul, J. (1992). A comparison of younger and older gay men's HIV risk-taking behaviors. *Journal of Acquired Immune Deficiency Syndrome, 5*:682-687.

van Gorder, D. & Henne, J. (1993, August). A Call for a New Generation of AIDS Prevention for Gay and Bisexual Men in San Francisco. San Francisco: San Francisco Department of Public Health.

von Aarburg, H-P. (1996, September). Sexualität zwischen psychohygienischer Fitness und Rausch in Deutsche AIDS-Hilfe. Riskomanagement: Aspekte der Primärprävention von HIV/AIDS. *Archiv für Sozialpolitik*: 31-41.

Williams, J. B. W., Rabkin, J. G., Remein, R. H., Gorman, J. M., & Ehrhardt, A. A. (1991). Multidisciplinary baseline assessment of homosexual men with and without HIV infection. *Archives of General Psychiatry, 48*: 124-30.

Context Is Everything: Thoughts on Effective HIV Prevention and Gay Men in the United States

Eric Rofes, MA

SUMMARY. As we approach the third decade of AIDS, HIV prevention in the United States confronts expanding public concern about continuing infections among gay men. This paper provides a brief history of HIV prevention efforts among gay men in the United States, as well as a succinct analysis of its successes and failures. By focusing on lessons learned from work in the 1980s–as well as lessons which have not yet been learned–the author suggests future directions in HIV prevention for gay men which emphasize critical analysis of epidemiological trends, and countering the merging of gay identity with HIV infection. Supporting men to gain greater authority and responsibility for their sexual community-building and redevelopment is necessary for lowering the infection rate among successive generations of gay men. *[Article copies available for a fee from The Haworth Document Delivery Service: 1-800-342-9678. E-mail address: getinfo@haworthpressinc.com]*

In many countries, HIV prevention work with gay men was pulled together quickly and chaotically in the 1980s by a socially isolated, politically-scapegoated population whose members were, for the most part, deeply closeted in their work lives and invisible or marginalized in their communities of origin. In the US, gay men rapidly moved–in five short years–from denial to shock to terror to action. My comments here focus on the gay experience of AIDS in the United States.

Gay men in hard-hit American cities developed an understanding of AIDS as crisis. This crisis model reflected our experiences as we searched our stomachs for purple spots, watched our sex lives shift from places of pleasure and comfort to places of fear and dread, and opened our weekly gay papers to dozens of obituaries of handsome men with whom we had built community, danced, or tricked.

Our prevention focus was aimed at keeping men safe from what seemed like a lethal syndrome which we knew little about. Hence, we aimed to:

- Get information out as rapidly as it became available.
- Design interventions to get men to use condoms all the time in anal sex.
- Change community norms about sexual practices, drug use, and involvement in community life. This would mean spurring stronger involvement in volunteerism, encouraging a critical consciousness about drug use and sexual risk, and supporting the development of community leaders.

It's easy to look back at this time critically without acknowledging the miracles of the period: Programs were developed even before government funds became available; a diverse population–wracked by internal bickering and torn by racism–managed to keep working together; and, despite a powerful anti-gay, anti-sex, backlash from the theocratic right, gay men did not go back into the closet, but came out *en masse* to develop care and prevention programs for our many communities.

LESSONS LEARNED

The hard lessons we learned from the '80s include:

1. We need to take seriously the differences within the population we call *gay men.* What works for affluent white gay men may not work for gay men who are first generation Latino immigrants. What works for educated, middle class African-American gay men may not work for African-American gay men living in poverty. What works for 40-year-olds may not work for 20-year-olds . . . or 60-year-olds, for that matter (Hunter, 1994; Mason, 1995; Peterson, 1995; Peterson et al., 1995).

2. A population with a long history of victimization by government officials, medical doctors, scientific researchers, and media personnel will not easily and quickly see these sectors as trustworthy partners in prevention (Patton, 1985). Our communities must have ownership of HIV/STD prevention, in word as well as deed. We must lead it.
3. Sex is a core part of our gay male identity and culture and telling men not to have sex will not work. Programs which judge men with multiple partners or men with a taste for so-called *kinky sex* will lose the confidence of the community (Turner, 1997; Watney, 1994).

UNLEARNED LESSONS

There are also lessons which we did not learn from the 1980s but need to:

1. Context is everything in HIV/STD prevention. By designing urban prevention programs for gay men based on cognitive-behavioral models, we were responding to the authentic experience of crisis dominating the 1980s. The context shifted by the 1990s, making these models less appropriate. Prevention for gay men in epicenter cities has rarely acknowledged these shifts and has failed to embrace sociocultural models which enjoy great success throughout much of the Western world. For example, in 1997 most U.S. prevention projects still refused to utilize *negotiated safety,* a prevention strategy adopted in several countries (like Australia and the United Kingdom) which is aimed at gay men who want to consider not using condoms in their primary relationships, yet maintain condom use with casual partners.[1] In refusing to apply negotiated safety and similar strategies, the American projects pretend to be taking the moral high road, continuing the crisis-driven push to *use a condom every time*, despite studies which show that 25-40% of gay men fail to do so (AIDS Action Committee, 1991; Kelly et al., 1992; Whyte et al., 1997).
2. There is not one gay male epidemic, but many different gay male HIV/AIDS epidemics. The gay event of AIDS has been defined by the experience of gay-identified men in San Francisco and New York. We see this in mainstream movies, plays, and books. Yet AIDS has happened very differently for gay men in rural Oregon than for gay men in San Francisco. Also, many young gay men in San Francisco do not experience AIDS as crisis–not because they are young, or in denial, or drunk–but because their everyday experience of AIDS in San Francisco is dramatically different now from

what it was for my generation in 1985. Our programs for gay men rarely take seriously the different geographic, generational, and class-based gay male epidemics.
3. Our communities cease to listen if we treat them with disrespect, disgust, or deception. We told gay men they must use condoms every time, treating their desires as expendable, dismissing the meanings many men find in being penetrated and in receiving another man's semen inside them. HIV prevention educators in San Francisco disrespected the central position of specific sex acts in many men's identities and treated anal sex with disgust and queer bodies as sites to be colonized. While claiming to *empower*, we used methods of manipulation, policing, subtle guilt-tripping, and out-right shaming. For example, some HIV prevention leaders have encouraged men to interrupt others who are having unprotected sex in public (Fera & Blankenship, 1993). Another example are the many U.S. support groups which have focused on prevention. While claiming to be *non-judgmental* and *peer-based*, many have, in fact, recommended that facilitators use group persuasion techniques to promote collective negative responses to incidents of unprotected sex.[2] These sorts of approaches have created the community we inhabit today: Cities populated by increasing numbers of gay men who distrust, disbelieve, and do not practice the guidelines set forth by our own organizations (Dangerous Bedfellows, 1997).

I believe our work in prevention needs to regularly take a deep breath in order to reexamine its theoretical foundations and to take a searching and fearless look at whether our methods are respectful, honest, and appropriate to the changing context of various gay HIV epidemics. Crisis-driven behavior change and cognitive approaches so popular in public health may no longer be effective in an epidemic approaching its third decade.

Currently, HIV/STD prevention for gay men is at a crossroads. We can continue fine-tuning traditional interventions focused on providing individual gay men with information, motivation, and skills. Or we can acknowledge the complexity of sexuality, trusting and supporting gay men to truly manage their own risk. Why does it seem staggering that, currently, a man would allow himself to be penetrated without protection? Why do we believe that swallowing semen is something gay men will be able to give up for the rest of their lives? We can pathologize these men as drunk, dumb, or self-destructive, or we can understand them as trying to develop strategies to continue practices which offer a core of meaning to their identities and to their lives as a whole, supporting them in these efforts.

HIV prevention must assume a broad mission focused on social and cultural interventions which assist gay men in creating meaningful lives that are worth living. Rather than asking "How can we help gay men to stop unsafe sex?" we might ask, "How can we help gay men to create lives which are worth living?" Rather than inquiring "How can we use peer-pressure to intervene in both private and public sex acts?" we can ask, "What can our community offer to gay men which is affirming and life-sustaining?"

FUTURE DIRECTIONS IN HIV PREVENTION

I think the recent Consensus Statement of the National Institutes of Health regarding HIV prevention might be improved by expanding the notion of HIV prevention so as to tackle social and cultural questions which ultimately determine infection rates. For example:

1. How can we prevention workers analyze shifts in the epidemic carefully and thoroughly? How can we avoid buying the simplistic and quick analysis of journalists? An example of this lack of care and thoroughness are the strong statements from some prevention leaders that the hope created by protease inhibitors has resulted in increased unsafe sex. Such comments have been made in spite of having, as yet, no data to support this claim. I wonder if current upswings in unprotected sex in some areas may be attributed–not to hearing discussions on protease inhibitors or reading articles about the *end of AIDS* and deciding to keep the condom in the wallet–but to being held hostage by a terrorized psyche for over a dozen years and no longer feeling anything at all.
2. How do we lift the imprint of AIDS off gay identity? The merging of *gay* with *AIDS* leads many young gay men to believe infection is inevitable (Van Gorder, 1993). We need to seriously consider ways to separate AIDS from gay identity. For example, we need to encourage community celebrations focused on building spirit and enjoying life which do not begin with a moment of silence or with draping panels of the Quilt over our heads.
3. How can we support gay men to have greater authority and responsibility for their sex? This means we need to seriously examine our educational methods. Why does a community which consistently draws parallels between itself and social change movements to liberate racial minorities choose, as models for HIV prevention, corporate marketing strategies rather than educational theories developed to empower oppressed groups? Gay men are depicted as consumers

to be pitched specific marketing messages, as if our erotic desires have so much in common with consumer urges for *Pepsi Cola*, a *Big Mac*, or *Jeep Cherokees*. Dialogue and reflection are superseded by seven-second sound bites and four-word slogans on the sides of buses. After a dozen years of such efforts, gay men may be more familiar with catchy prevention slogans which bombard us on billboards and T-shirts and bus shelters than with the physiology of our own penises. We might focus instead on true empowerment-based models of education, as pioneered by Paulo Freire, for the next generation of prevention work (Freire, 1970).

For most populations of gay men, what will make the greatest difference is not new posters or new messages. Prevention must support gay men as we reinvent our identities and create communities beyond suffering and cultures beyond crisis. A valuable agenda would focus on the self-conscious reconstruction of gay communities after the avalanche of AIDS hit. New HIV prevention efforts must be redefined to be as much about creating community centers and invigorating social networks as it is about safe sex guidelines.

Would the US government ever fund community-building for queer men as some governments of other Western industrialized countries do? The reader may wonder: What planet does this guy live on? What recommendations can I take away from this madman?

First, HIV prevention theorists and program developers need to invite researchers from other disciplines into the discussion. We have talked about this for a long time, but too often in AIDS we talk within narrow behaviorist disciplines. And in doing this, we all lose. We need to take seriously the *new thinking* on prevention pioneered by psychologists like Walt Odets, sociologists like Gary Dowsett, anthropologists such as Ralph Bolton, and cultural studies scholars like Cindy Patton.

Second, we need to think of prevention as more than brochures and lists of do's and don'ts. We need to consider social interventions and big picture, long-term issues, rather than simple individual-based approaches. We should focus on men being in dialogue with each other, not as passive receptacles waiting to receive our directives and wisdom.

Third, we should integrate community building as a central part of HIV prevention. This pertains to all our communities and, in fact, is something we can learn from other communities' attempts, for example, to stop teenage pregnancy or to encourage kids to stop using drugs. Context is everything, so community-building must be central to our work.

CONCLUSION

I make these recommendations because AIDS is not enough. Community cannot be defined by disease. Meaning in life will not come from an epidemic without context. People need more, want more, and deserve more. In the 1980s, AIDS provided gay men with direction and purpose, but as the epidemic proved more tenacious than expected, gay male identity, community, and sexuality merged with a syndrome of viral infection and opportunistic disease. Life narrowed incredibly, until the self-images of men were defined, in large part, by the presence or absence of a microscopic virus in our bloodstream.

This is no way to build community. It is no way to live a life. We need a vision of community that neither denies the realities of AIDS nor is held hostage to its demands. It is time for prevention to place AIDS in a position of balance in gay community life. The lives of gay men must integrate the realities of an ongoing epidemic, while providing a broader, life-affirming agenda.

If we as gay men are to protect ourselves effectively from HIV, we must have lives which we deeply believe are worth living. If we hope to see the powerful reemergence of gay communities as vital entities offering sustenance and meaning, we must shift our resources and talents to this effort. If gay community is to be more than a commodities market, more than a mass culture of crisis, a concerted effort to redesign, re-energize, and regenerate collective life must be initiated. This is the new direction of HIV/STD prevention for gay men.

NOTES

1. In a paper published in 1997, the leading United States AIDS prevention research center suggested negotiated safety might be a useful technique for groups to consider. See Hoff et al., 1997.

2. This was discussed explicitly in the peer facilitator trainings of STOP AIDS/Los Angeles during 1987-1988 when I oversaw the program at the Los Angeles Gay and Lesbian Community Services Center.

BIBLIOGRAPHY

AIDS Action Committee (1981). *A Survey of AIDS-Related Knowledge, Attitudes and Behaviors Among Gay and Bisexual Men in Greater Boston.* Boston: AIDS Action Committee.

Bolton, R. (1992). AIDS and promiscuity: Muddles in the models of HIV prevention. *Medical Anthropology, 14*: 145-223.

Bolton, R. (1992). Mapping terra incognita: Sex research for AIDS prevention: An urgent agenda for the 1990s. In G. Herdt and S. Lindenbaum (Eds.), *The Time of AIDS: Social Analysis, Theory, and Method*. Newbury Park, CA: Sage.

Bolton, R., Vincke, J., Mak, R., & Dennehy, E. (1992). Alcohol and risky sex: In search of an elusive connection. *Medical Anthropology, 14*: 323-363.

Brummelhuis, H. ten, & Herdt, G. (1995). *Culture and Sexual Risk: Anthropological Perspectives on AIDS*. Amsterdam: Gordon and Breach.

Carballo-Dieguez, A., & Dolezal, C. (1994). Contrasting types of Puerto Rican men who have sex with men (MSM). *Journal of Psychology & Human Sexuality, 6*(4): 41-67.

Colter, E. (1997). Discernibly turgid: Safer sex and public policy. In Dangerous Bedfellows (Eds.), *Policing Public Sex*. Boston: South End Press.

Connell, R.W., Crawford, J., Dowsett, G. W., Kippax, S., Sinnott, V., Rodden, P., Berg, R., Baxter, D., & Watson, L. (1990). Danger and context: Unsafe anal sexual practice among homosexual and bisexual men in the AIDS crisis. *Australian and New Zealand Journal of Sociology, 26*(2): 187-208.

Dangerous Bedfellows (1997). *Policing Public Sex*. Boston: South End Press.

de Zwart, O. (1995). The structure and meaning of anal sex among gay men. Proceedings of AIDS in Europe–The Behavioral Aspects: European Conference on Methods and Results of Psycho-Social AIDS Research. Berlin: Sigma.

Dowsett, G. (1996). *Practicing Desire: Homosexual Sex in the Era of AIDS*. Stanford, CA: Stanford University Press.

Fera, J., & Blankenship, W. (1993, November 24). It's Not Acceptable, in 1993 . . . *[San Francisco] Bay Area Reporter*, 6.

Freire, P. (1970). *The Pedagogy of the Oppressed*. [trans. Myra Bergman Ramos]. New York: Continuum.

Gold, R. (1995). Why We Need to Rethink AIDS Education for Gay Men? Plenary address at the Second International Conference on AIDS' Impact: Biopsychosocial Aspects of HIV Infection, 7-10 July, Brighton, U.K.

Gold, R., Skinner, M., & Ross, M. (1994). Unprotected anal intercourse in HIV-infected and non-HIV-infected gay men. *Journal of Sex Research, 31*: 59-77.

Herdt, G., & Boxer, A. (1991). Ethnographic issues in the study of AIDS. *Journal of Sex Research, 28*(2): 171-187.

Hoff, C., Stall, R., Paul, J., Acress, M., Daigle, D., Phillips, K., Kegeles, S., Jinich, S., Ekstrand, M., & Coates, T. J. (1997). Differences in sexual behavior among HIV discordant and concordant gay men in primary relationships. *Journal of Acquired Immune Deficiency Syndromes and Human Retrovirology, 14*: 72-78.

Hunter, J., & Schaecher, R. (1994). AIDS prevention for lesbian, gay, and bisexual adolescents. *Families in Society: The Journal of Contemporary Human Services*, 346-354.

Johnson, W. (1995). *HIV negative: How the uninfected are affected by AIDS*. New York: Insight Books.

Kelly, J. A., Murphy, D. A., Roffman, R. A., Solomon, L. J., Winett, R. A., Stevenson, L. Y., Koob, J. J., Ayotte, D. R., Flynn, B. S., Desideratro, L. L. et al. (1992). Acquired Immonodeficiency Syndrome/Human Immunodeficiency

Virus risk behavior among gay men in small cities. *Archives of Internal Medicine, 152*: 2293-2297.

Keogh, P. (1996, July). HIV Prevention Amongst Gay Men: Personal Strategies and Community Responses. Paper presented for Deutche AIDS-Hilfe Satellite Session, Vancouver, Canada.

Kerkhof, M. P. N., de Zwart, O., & Sandfort, T. (1996). *Viewed from Behind: Anal Sex in the AIDS Era*. Utrecht: Utrecht University, Gay and Lesbian Studies.

King, E. (1993). *Safety in Numbers: Safer Sex and Gay Men*. New York: Routledge.

Kippax, S. et al. (1995). Predictors of unprotected male-to-male anal intercourse with casual partners in a national sample. *Australian Journal of Public Health, 19*(2): 132-138.

Mason, H. R. C., Marks, G., Simoni, J. M., Ruiz, M. S., & Richardson, J. L. (1995). Culturally sanctioned secrets? Latino men's nondisclosure of HIV infection to family, friends and lovers. *Health Psychology, 14*(1): 6-12.

Odets, W. (1996). Why we stopped doing primary prevention for gay men in 1985. In Dangerous Bedfellows (Ed.), *Policing Public Sex*. Boston: South End Press.

Odets, W. (1995). *In the Shadow of the Epidemic: Being HIV-Negative in the Age of AIDS*. Durham, NC: Duke University Press.

Patton, C. (1985). *Sex and Germs: The Politics of AIDS*. Boston: South End Press.

Patton, C. (1990). *Inventing AIDS*. New York: Routledge.

Patton, C. (1996). *Fatal Advice: How Safe-Sex Education Went Wrong*. Durham, NC: Duke University Press.

Peterson, J. L. (1995). AIDS-related risks and same sex behavior among African-American men. In G. Herek & B. Greene (Eds.), *AIDS, Identity and Community*. Thousand Oaks, CA: Sage. 85-104.

Peterson, J. L., Coates, T. J., Catania, J. A., Hilliard, B., Middleton, L., & Hearst, N. (1995). Help-seeking for AIDS high-risk sexual behavior among gay and bisexual African-American men. *AIDS Education and Prevention, 7*(1): 1-9.

Rofes, E. (1996). *Reviving the Tribe: Regenerating Gay Men's Sexuality and Culture in the Ongoing Epidemic*. Binghamton, NY: The Haworth Press, Inc.

Rofes, E. (1998). *Dry Bones Breathe: Gay Men Creating Post-AIDS Identities and Cultures*. Binghamton, NY: The Haworth Press, Inc.

Rosser, B. R. S. (1991). The effects of using fear in public AIDS education on the behaviour of homosexually active men. *Journal of Psychology and Human Sexuality, 4*(3): 123-134.

Rosser, B. R. S., Coleman, E., & Ohmans, P. (1993). Safer sex maintenance and reduction of unsafe sex among homosexually active men: A new therapeutic approach. *Health Education Research: Theory and Practice, 8*(1): 19-34.

Savage, D. (1997, January 16). Life After AIDS. *The Stranger* [Seattle, WA].

Turner, D. (1997). *Risky Sex: Gay Men and HIV Prevention*. New York: Columbia.

van Gorder, D. (Ed.) (1993, August). A call for a new generation of AIDS prevention for gay and bisexual men in San Francisco. San Francisco Department of Health.

Warner, M. (1995, January 31). Why gay men are having risky sex. *The Village Voice.*
Watney, S. (1987). *Policing Desire: Pornography, AIDS, and the Media.* Minneapolis: University of Minnesota.
Watney, S. (1994). *Practices of Freedom: Selected Writings on HIV/AIDS.* Durham, NC: Duke University Press.
Whyte, J., Green, E., Polansky, M., & Bartlett, C. (1997). Men's survey report: Assessing the knowledge, attitudes, beliefs, and behaviors regarding HIV. Philadelphia: AIDS Information Network.
Wright, M. (1998). Beyond Risk Factors: Trends in European Safer Sex Research. *New International Directions in HIV Prevention for Gay and Bisexual Men.* Binghamton, NY: The Haworth Press, Inc.

The Impact of New Advances in Treatment on HIV Prevention: Implications of the XI International AIDS Conference on Future Prevention Directions

B. R. Simon Rosser, PhD, MPH

SUMMARY. This paper examines the impact of new advances in treatment on HIV prevention targeting men who have sex with men. A period of uncertainty, with new questions and complex issues, is predicted. HIV prevention is rapidly changing, a result of such factors as: the introduction of protease inhibitors and other new medications, improvements in HIV detection and testing technologies, the confusion about sub-detectable viral load levels, funding dilemmas, divergence of rich and poor both within countries and between countries, anti-retroviral prophylaxis following occupational and possibly sexual exposure, and the emergence of black markets. The emergence of *the new AIDS poor* and the changing epidemic profile of HIV will mean significant challenges for AIDS Service Organizations (ASOs). The behavioral labelling of men who have sex with men and the focus of prevention on anal intercourse impacts our sense of gay, bisexual and queer identities. The challenges of this new HIV prevention era: for prevention workers to become familiar with new information about medications and virology, for social science research to become more interdisciplinary, and for information dissemination to become more efficient and broad. We have entered a period of many new questions with few answers, necessitating HIV prevention to become informed, flexible and united. *[Article copies available for a fee from The Haworth Document Delivery Service: 1-800-342-9678. E-mail address: getinfo@haworthpressinc.com]*

While the XI International Conference on AIDS (Vancouver) and the 18th National Lesbian and Gay Health Conference and AIDS Forum (Seattle) provided a wealth of new information to participants, new questions about the impact of these advances on HIV prevention emerge. This report summarizes some of the specific issues identified by a caucus at the Seattle conference convened to address these concerns.

At the XI International Conference on AIDS, in both the basic and clinical science tracks, a number of new discoveries and important advances were reported that appear to be making significant in-roads in our understanding and treatment of HIV. Scientists left expressing cautious optimism about new developments. Although many of these developments are experimental, and others are in design, development or testing phases, they raise important questions for HIV prevention, for our understanding of safer sex, for persons living with HIV/AIDS and for the wider gay, lesbian, bisexual and transgender (GLBT) communities.

HIV As a Long-Term Manageable Illness. Exciting new possibilities of HIV/AIDS becoming a long-term treatable disease have emerged. Because of these possibilities, HIV prevention information will need to change in ways we don't yet fully understand. We need to prepare for a period of uncertainty where we will have many questions raising incomplete answers. What is clear is that previous simplistic slogans will not be adequate to address the increasingly complex situations for HIV prevention brought about by advances in viral understanding, detection, and treatment. What is also clear, is that the HIV prevention paradigms currently in use will need to change.

Hope in a Cure: Impact on Prevention. Psychologically, caucus participants wondered how the new *hope* raised by these advances will affect people's safer sex decision-making. Even if notions of a "cure" are still some time away, what effect will "long-term management" have on risk behavior and relapse? In communities most affected by HIV, to what extent will we dare to hope, when previous treatments turned out less effective than initially expected? Because HIV prevention volunteers and peer educators are often conduits of knowledge to those most affected, prevention personnel will need education, first, regarding advances in virology and treatments, and second, in the impact of these on HIV prevention. We need to establish clear mechanisms for education now, if we are to avoid chaos, confusion and misunderstandings related to these developments.

New HIV Testing Methodologies. New *testing methodologies* are emerging, including saliva, dry blood, and home HIV testing. While of enormous assistance to those with fears of blood, the saliva test has the potential to re-ignite public concerns and misinformation about saliva transmission, especially in those with marginal access to education. With home-testing, we need to address how to best assist compulsive AIDS testers to manage their compulsivity. Under development, test kits that will yield immediate test results could assist HIV prevention enormously. In the not too distant future, instant HIV tests may become to sex what breathalysers are to driving under the influence. We need to anticipate the effects such new technologies will have on safer sex decision-making and practices.

The Impact of Viral Load and New Medications on HIV Prevention. Clearly, the face of HIV prevention is changing. For example, *protease inhibitors* raise the promise for at least some people with HIV of lowering *viral load* to sub-detectable levels. How will this affect transmission and our beliefs about who are most at risk of transmitting HIV? New questions arise. What risk will persons with sub-detectable levels of virus be of transmitting HIV? Carefully designed studies are urgently needed to examine this question. In HIV prevention, will we continue to consider all HIV positives at risk of transmitting HIV or will the new population at risk of transmission be those who are not under treatment, and those not tested? Similarly, many researchers at Vancouver stressed the concern that as treatment regimens become complex, unprotected sex among HIV positives could lead to *viral mutation* and *drug resistant* strains of HIV. What does this mean for secondary prevention efforts targeting persons with HIV/AIDS? It appears we may need a new education campaign to address the specific implications of new medications for HIV positives. Both prevention education and research is needed to pursue important questions relating medication adherence and transmission risk.

Funding Challenges. Some of the most difficult dilemmas we must face relate to *funding* and the disbursement of limited resources. What proportion of resources will be allocated to treatment and what to prevention will become even more difficult to determine. How these decisions will be made and by whom is critical, and GLBT persons need to ensure our voice and concerns are included. There is great potential for our communities to become split: between those advocating service provision and those prevention, between people with HIV and those negative, and between those who can access resources and those who cannot. Already some states in the U.S. have shifted prevention funds to fund new medications. Another identified danger is the tendency to prematurely downsize prevention efforts during a period of optimism regarding treatments. As new interventions necessitate review of existing resource allocation, how do we balance the importance of providing access to treatments for those infected with the cost-effectiveness of prevention efforts to support people remaining negative?

As *new medications* develop, it would appear important to study the sexual behavioral implications of these on communities most at risk. There are exciting new possibilities of medications preventing infection, including discussion of an after-possible-exposure-prevention pill, the development of vaginal microbicides to prevent transmission, vaccine development and treatment to immediately suppress viral replication in the newly-infected. While not yet developed, these new technologies may take us beyond reliance on condoms and non-penetrative sex to prevent HIV, but in turn raise completely new challenges for prevention. In the interim, as a high risk population, homosexually-active men are likely to be asked to participate in studies of promising but unproven technologies. As a community, we need to discuss now to what degree and under what circumstances we want to be part of these developments. As *new technologies* to prevent transmission are under development, it will be important to ensure that technologies to address homosexual transmission are given adequate priority.

Forgotten Populations and the New Poor. At the caucus, concern was expressed for frequently overlooked populations. For *transgendered persons*, studies may be needed to assess the interaction effects of new medications and hormones. Just as women need to assert their inclusion in studies on HIV, so transgendered persons may need to assert the importance of their being integrated into protocols. While several speakers at Vancouver expressed concern that only those living in resource rich countries will be able to afford new medications, we also need to think about the poor, minorities, homeless, women and others in our own communities who are less likely to gain access to treatments. It is difficult to predict how the emergence of life-sustaining treatments may impact the risk behavior of those who perceive themselves shut out from access to such treatments. As HIV is ultimately a global concern, those GLBT communities in *resource rich* countries may be called on to champion the needs of those in *resource poor* countries. Finally, in the rush and hope of new treatments, those not able to tolerate these treatments must not be forgotten. ASOs need to be prepared to assist those whose hopes were raised only to have them dashed once again.

Post-HIV Exposure Prophylaxis. At the conference, protocols for taking *anti-retrovirals* following *occupational exposure* were announced. But should health providers be the only ones to have access to these, and should we be advocating for similar protocols following sexual exposure? In either regard, we need to examine the impact of these protocols on current safer sexual and drug behavior among those at risk. This raises the perplexing issue of *patterns of risk behavior*, namely, if such medications are made available, will some people begin to rely on *anti-retrovirals as prophylaxis*, and if so, what will be the long-term effects of repeated interventions? To what extent will HIV negative people who relapse seek out limited HIV treatments as prophylaxis, and what long-term effects will this have on drug efficacy?

Indirect Effects of HIV Medication Developments. As new medications develop, often indirect yet predictable patterns follow. To the degree that new treatments are limited, underground *black markets* may follow, and with that, greater variation in medication use. We can expect the emergence of *"desperate"* people, that is, those who are denied direct access to new treatments and who will do anything to access these medications. This variation in *medication adherence* and underground dispensing has important implications for viral resistance.

Impact on AIDS Service Organizations. As long-term survival becomes more pronounced, *AIDS Service Organizations* (ASOs) face new challenges. For some PWAs, the reversal of serious debilitations that until recently were seen as symptomatic of decline, is posing new issues. *Rehabilitation* may be needed to assist some of those previously on disability to re-enter the job market. Others have become the *"new AIDS poor,"* those who once enjoyed a good standard of living, but who may have lost all economic security to AIDS, only to now be given a second chance to begin again. Still others, especially those with enduring disabilities, may choose *not* to avail themselves of life-prolonging medications. The need to respect choices and address the difficult ethical dilemmas raised by life-sustaining treatments is required.

Impact of Prevention Research. Behavioral research on HIV has given us new and complex ways of defining our communities. *Men who have sex with men (MSM)*, *males who have sex with males*, *homosexually-active men*, *sex between men*, and *male-male sex* are all behavioral labels introduced by HIV prevention. We need to study how these new definitions are changing our sense of gay, bisexual and queer identities, while reinforcing principally the sexual aspect of our lives. Do these *behavioral labels* provide a new closet, where men can avoid identifying with their behavior and thus do these descriptors themselves become impediments to people coming out?

Impact of New Information. We can anticipate drug companies continuing to introduce highly complex and, thus, potentially confusing *new information* about new medications. While in the past, the time taken to have new drugs approved meant that drug companies had time to work with and prepare the community, new fast-track licensing methods necessitate development of stream-lined information dissemination. The communities most affected by HIV need to develop more efficient means of working with drug companies so that the impact of new medications on prevention can be predicted and addressed. We need to be mindful of the *ethical obligations* that pharmaceutical companies have to examine the impact of new technology on risk behaviors, and our own ethical obligations to be *active participants* in prevention and service delivery. We need to examine our role or roles as GLBT communities and ASOs, so as to maximize the benefits of these developments and minimize confusion and other negative effects that may occur. Above all, we must never become part of the problem, but remain committed to furthering solutions.

Guiding the Way. The caucus identified the following potential responses to assist HIV prevention. The need for *social science research* in many disciplines–including ethics, behavioral medicine, psychology, sociology, interdisciplinary research and systemic research–focus on these new questions if we are to proceed in an informed and intelligent way. A *statement of guiding principles*, similar to the Denver Principles, may be needed to provide consistency. *Symposia* specifically addressing the HIV prevention impact of these new technologies are needed. Since the aim of these symposia is to address the effects of new technologies and treatments, the pharmaceutical companies may be appropriate funding sources for these. *Community forums, town hall meetings* and other *venues of discussion* may be needed to help the GLBT communities participate, disseminate and strategize our responses to these developments. *Discussion papers* and *pamphlets* which address these questions would help standardize information and assist community members to be informed.

CONCLUSION

Clearly, we have many new questions that are critical and few answers or processes in place to assist us to navigate this new territory. Both individually and communally, the challenges are clear. We must become informed, flexible, and united in our commitments to both prevention and treatment. We need to develop new strategies, paradigms, and community processes that will enable us to yield maximum benefit from these developments both for treatment and prevention. And above all, we must remain united in the fight against HIV and in our commitment to an informed approach to HIV prevention.

The Impact of New Treatments and Other Trends on HIV Prevention for Gay and Bisexual Men in the United States: Observations from the 19th National Lesbian and Gay Health Association Conference

B. R. Simon Rosser, PhD, MPH
Michael T. Wright, LICSW, MS

SUMMARY. This paper details how HIV prevention workers in the United States are being impacted by advances in HIV/AIDS treatments and a changing HIV prevention paradigm. Approximately sixty participants attending the 1997 National Lesbian and Gay Health Conference and AIDS Forum in Atlanta, GA, provided observations about how HIV prevention targeting men who have sex with men is changing in the United States. While new treatments may be the most noticeable change impacting HIV prevention, radical change due to the synergistic effects of several factors, not only recent medical advances, is seen as propelling a paradigm shift. Twelve challenges were identified and suggestions for facilitating progress in the changing

---

[Haworth co-indexing entry note]: "The Impact of New Treatments and Other Trends on HIV Prevention for Gay and Bisexual Men in the United States: Observations from the 19th National Lesbian and Gay Health Association Conference." Rosser, B. R. Simon, and Michael T. Wright. Co-published simultaneously in *Journal of Psychology & Human Sexuality* (The Haworth Press, Inc.) Vol. 10, No. 3/4, 1998, pp. 151-158; and: *New International Directions in HIV Prevention for Gay and Bisexual Men* (ed: Michael T. Wright, B. R. Simon Rosser, and Onno de Zwart) The Haworth Press, Inc., 1998, pp. 151-158; and: *New International Directions in HIV Prevention for Gay and Bisexual Men* (ed: Michael T. Wright, B. R. Simon Rosser, and Onno de Zwart) Harrington Park Press, an imprint of The Haworth Press, Inc., 1998, pp. 151-158. Single or multiple copies of this article are available for a fee from The Haworth Document Delivery Service [1-800-342-9678, 9:00 a.m. - 5:00 p.m. (EST). E-mail address: getinfo@haworthpressinc.com].

© 1998 by The Haworth Press, Inc. All rights reserved.

paradigm enumerated. The future of HIV prevention is discussed. *[Article copies available for a fee from The Haworth Document Delivery Service: 1-800-342-9678. E-mail address: getinfo@haworthpressinc.com]*

A critical but under-studied area of HIV prevention is how communities at risk for infection are impacted by advances in treatment. In addition, other trends taking place at the organizational level of AIDS service organizations often go unobserved in the usual HIV/AIDS research and prevention literature. Two meetings were held in 1996 and 1997 at the annual conference of the National Lesbian and Gay Health Association (National Lesbian and Gay Health Conference/National HIV/AIDS Forum) to explore, from the perspective of a diverse group of practitioners in the field, the impact of medical advances on HIV prevention in the United States for men who have sex with men (MSM). Also discussed at these meetings were general trends in prevention and education (see Rosser, this volume).

This article reports the results of the follow-up meeting conducted in 1997 in Atlanta. One year after the first announcements of the new treatments, participants were able to reflect concretely on their experiences of doing prevention work in light of medical advances as well as on other developments in the field from their frontline perspective.

METHODS

Approximately 60 participants attended the session, which was facilitated by the two authors. Those in attendance were all active in the field of HIV prevention, including male and female health professionals, paraprofessionals, researchers, activists, and others who serve and/or identify with the gay and bisexual male communities. With the exception of two Europeans, all participants were American. The session began with a review of the previous year's observations to establish continuity, then participants broke into small groups to identify the impact of new treatments and other developments on their work over the last year. Participants were asked to identify up to three *major challenges you face in your work because of the changing paradigm.* The results of these small groups were reported back into the larger group. Participants were then asked to formulate how we can further progress in HIV prevention, given the changing landscape.

RESULTS

Participants' observations of the challenges to HIV prevention in light of the changing paradigm are reported in Table 1. Table 2 denotes how

TABLE 1. Challenges Facing HIV Prevention in Light of the Changing Paradigm *(N = 60 HIV prevention personnel targeting MSM)*

1. The efficacy and success of new treatments have been a focus. The complexity, difficulty, and failure of treatments have been underestimated in the gay/bisexual community.

2. The need for consistent, accurate, and understandable information about new treatments and virology has increased. Access to treatment information is a concern.

3. With the emergence of new treatments, the sense of urgency in HIV prevention is waning, both in the general public and among gay/bisexual men.

4. Media presentations and perceptions have changed, with articles about Magic Johnson being "cured" adding to public misconceptions about undetectable viral load.

5. Funding for HIV prevention appears under threat as funds have been siphoned towards treatment, and AIDS has been "downgraded" in importance.

6. There is a sense of exhaustion among prevention workers and a public wish for this epidemic to be over. The advances in treatment are mistaken by some to mean we no longer have a problem. People have moved into their "comfort zone," becoming less open to HIV prevention.

7. In the "post-AIDS" era, there has begun a dismantling of the structures which were built by and for middle-class, white gay/bisexual men. There is a growing need to address race and class specific issues as the epidemic changes. In some agencies, there is the fear of losing "turf" and jobs, as HIV is increasingly identified as having moved beyond the adult gay/bisexual community.

8. Important cultural barriers to HIV prevention exist. The epidemic in white men who have sex with men is often presented as being over, while the epidemic among men of color is increasing. This can lead to further segmentation of gay communities by ethnicity.

9. The issue of post-exposure prophylaxis is complex. While the medical community appears quick to make available such treatment for fellow health professionals who incur needle-stick, they have been slow to offer similar assistance to gay and bisexual men exposed sexually. Concerns regarding the promotion of viral resistance, replacing behavioral prevention with prophylaxis, and claims of homophobia are becoming confused in this discussion.

TABLE 1 (continued)

10. There have been many anecdotal reports of the effects of treatment on risk taking behavior; however, the evidence is inconclusive. To what degree men are increasing unsafe sex because of new treatments, and to what degree this is this year's "rationale" for unsafe sex is unknown. There is an urgent need for research to be undertaken, studying how the new treatments are changing both HIV positive and HIV negative men's safer sex behavior and decision making. Sexual behavior studies undertaken prior to the use of protease inhibitors may no longer provide valid estimates of actual behavior.

11. As new, more effective medications become available, there are growing ethical concerns about who is treated, and who makes that decision. For example, homeless men may be denied treatment, as they could be considered to present compliance risks.

12. AIDS Services organizations (ASOs) must be prepared to change. In many situations, ASOs may need to close, with HIV services being incorporated into larger structures which address broader issues of gay men's health.

TABLE 2. How to Facilitate Progress in HIV Prevention

A. Is the largest group of HIV-infected Americans, white gay men, being forgotten?

1. The needs of gay white men need to be delineated. While in most parts of the country, this group still comprises the largest number of Americans to become infected each year, services for this group are under threat of being discontinued. This is a dangerous tendency which should be resisted.

2. To date, gay white men have dominated HIV prevention work. As the epidemic profile changes, there are interesting challenges facing our community: How can we involve the missing voices (both gay men of color and lesbians). How can we avoid the "colonialization" by white, middle-class, middle-aged gay men of gay men of other ethnicities, ages, and classes? What happens to the white gay men who may have given years of their careers to this epidemic and now find themselves being asked to stand aside so that other voices can be heard? Should these men stand aside, and if so, how do we ensure that the experience of these men is not lost? These issues must be faced and discussed within the gay community.

3. How do gay white men play into structural homophobia by being too quick to downplay their own needs in the interest of supporting the demands of other groups? When should gay white men stop and challenge the trend to target resources towards "emerging populations" and away from their own experience and community? When will white gay men stand up for themselves?

B. *Targeting, not splitting, the gay community: Class, color, and serostatus.*

1. There is danger in separating white MSM from MSM of color. Progress in HIV prevention must resist the targeting of MSM which results in splintering the community.
2. HIV prevention has focused on racial issues, which minimizes the role class plays in fueling the epidemic. With changes in health care, there is a need to address the emergence of a new underclass and the effects of this on the epidemic.
3. As HIV submerges increasingly into the lower class, there is the danger of segmenting the gay community into class groups.
4. There need to be prevention messages for HIV positive men which are more clearly related to this group's lived experience. This needs to be done in such a way as to not divide the community by serostatus.

C. *HIV testing and intervention.*

1. Diagnosing and intervening during time of seroconversion is likely to become state-of-the-art treatment. We need to develop guidelines and protocols to facilitate this. This will require immediate result HIV tests and viral load estimates.
2. The role of testing needs to be re-thought, as new possibilities and challenges emerge. There is the possibility of a new consensus on the issue of testing.

D. *Effects of treatment on prevention.*

1. There is a danger in seeing protease inhibitors as the answer, rather than only one step in a series of developments. Effective treatments raise issues of access, and HIV prevention workers may find themselves playing increasing roles as advocates for the poor and under-represented.
2. We need to clarify goals of our work in light of new treatments. Is the primary goal to maintain people's serostatus as HIV negative or to advocate for quality of life issues for people undergoing treatment?

E. *HIV prevention or gay men's health.*

1. There is an urgent need to radically re-think HIV prevention targeting gay men. As the paradigms change, so too, our approaches to our work need to change.
2. HIV prevention agencies serving gay men may need to either integrate into other service structures or develop into gay men's health centers–otherwise they may face closure. There needs to be a focus on gay men's health beyond HIV. We need to reject a disease-specific approach and focus rather on underlying issues, causes, and factors related to illness. Community mobilization is likely to become more important.

TABLE 2 (continued)

F. Impact of Community Planning Groups on gay men's health agenda.

1. The community planning groups, established by the CDC, have revolutionized prevention planning. However, the power of these groups is being threatened by divisiveness as various target groups compete for funding. Because of representation issues, the gay voice within these groups has become less influential. There is a need for gay input at the national level to re-emerge. Otherwise, the danger is that all target groups will lose.

participants anticipate progress can be made in HIV prevention during this period of change. The tables were produced by grouping similar responses under headings reflecting common observations or issues.

Because of the emergence of new treatments, 1996-1997 may be a watershed year in the history of HIV/AIDS. But HIV prevention in the US is actually undergoing radical change due to the synergistic effects of several factors, not only recent medical advances. These factors include: protease inhibitors and the hope of HIV becoming a manageable, chronic illness; the importance of viral load in treating and managing HIV; the shift in HIV prevention from risk elimination to risk management and harm reduction; the changing dynamics of the nationally mandated community planning groups charged with resource allocation; changes in the gay, lesbian, bisexual, and transgender community (GLBT); the exhaustion of HIV prevention workers; and changing public opinion regarding HIV/AIDS.

As detailed in the tables, several of these factors impact psychologically to *down-grade* HIV in the minds of Americans in general, and of HIV prevention workers in particular. Participants stressed that although HIV remains the most serious, life-threatening epidemic impacting the gay community in the US, there is a growing lack of interest in the HIV prevention industry regarding this population. There is a need to counteract a current trend of funding treatment and services for other populations by taking monies away from prevention for men who have sex with men. Concern was expressed that prevention may be progressively dismantled for this population, particularly for white men.

DISCUSSION

Implications for Prevention. HIV prevention workers and researchers, as well as gay community representatives, are in a very difficult position. It is hardly *politically correct* to be fighting to keep resources within one's community—especially if that community is predominantly white men—when there are well-documented emerging epidemics in other communities. However, from an epidemiological perspective, in places where the majority of infections continue to be in the gay community, it makes sense for the majority of HIV prevention funding to target this population. The re-allocation and downgrading of prevention efforts to men who have sex with men seems premature.

Activism may be useful, particularly on the part of the community planning groups funded by the Centers for Disease Control and Prevention. These groups could join together, refusing to accept level-funding or reduced resources in an expanding epidemic, while demanding additional resources to target emerging populations. If steps are not taken, it appears that community planning groups are soon to become the vehicle for dividing target populations along race and socioeconomic lines, ultimately undermining effective, coordinated HIV prevention.

At the same time, there is widespread recognition that AIDS service structures cannot simply be defended and maintained in their current form. In the past twelve months, HIV prevention has changed dramatically, and participants identified the future of HIV prevention targeting men who have sex with men as involving even more radical change. In terms of gay men, there is strong interest in continuing HIV prevention within the context of gay health organizations and initiatives. This would mean reviving the gay health movement which was begun in the 1970s, but which has largely become synonymous with HIV programming since the outbreak of the AIDS epidemic. Within a more comprehensive gay health model, specific diseases would be targeted, such as HIV, but also the needs of particular under-served populations could be addressed, such as men of lower socioeconomic status.

There is a noticeable reluctance among prevention workers and researchers to move beyond traditional prevention to take on such issues as post-exposure prophylaxis and "instant" viral load testing. The former could potentially dramatically effect the incidence of illness, with the latter allowing for people to have direct information about their infectivity at the time of sexual encounter. Although still in the development stages, such issues need to be addressed proactively by HIV prevention workers and researchers if their work is to keep pace with the rapidly changing needs and interests of men who have sex with men.

Another topic needing consideration is the confusion regarding *undetectable* virus vs. *cure*. If low viral load does, in fact, lower transmissibility, this issue will need to be addressed when designing interventions for men who are HIV-positive. Both individually and communally, men who have sex with men may need to redefine risk and what are acceptable levels of risk. Again, this subject is quite different than traditional HIV prevention, but discussing this issue will be necessary so that men can make informed decisions.

Finally, providers of HIV services need to be able to define honestly and accurately the needs of their target groups versus the wishes of their own organization to survive. The transformation of HIV services will ultimately mean structural changes, including the integration of HIV prevention into other programs, changes in the definition of fundamental activities such as outreach, and a redefinition of priorities. Service providers are challenged to demonstrate the highest degree of flexibility so as to be proactive in creating new models as opposed to being recalcitrant players in a battle for funding.

CONCLUSION

The process of using the NLGHA conference to explore trends in HIV prevention in the U.S. for men who have sex with men is innovative, in that the gay community, particularly those members involved in the field of HIV prevention, are able to discuss the implications of the changing paradigm on their work and on the community as a whole. This format allows for a mutual interchange of information, both upward and downward, consistent with the gay community's demand to be equal partners with the scientific and medical communities in HIV prevention and treatment. We recommend that the National Lesbian and Gay Health Association continue this leadership role of assisting the gay community to anticipate, disseminate, and integrate advances in treatment and prevention of HIV. Given the unique national representation of the group assembled at these conferences, such meetings can become a dialog bridging researchers and frontline workers, providers and consumers, as well as HIV-positive and HIV-negative men so as to affect change in HIV prevention nationwide. Just as the HIV prevention movement in the US broke new ground in community health participation early in its history, the NLGHA caucus initiative may prove ground-breaking as a process for building understanding, leadership and unity in discerning and navigating new directions for HIV prevention in uncertain and complex times.

The meetings held at the 1996 and 1997 conferences make clear that the field of HIV for men who have sex with men in the U.S. is rapidly changing. The challenge to prevention workers and researchers is to respond flexibly and proactively so as to design effective and responsive programs for the future.

Authors' Notes

Susan Beardsell was a Senior Research Fellow with Sigma Research where she was the principle researcher on a variety of projects including Social and Psychological Issues in HIV Testing and studies of Genitourinary Medicine Clinics and Needle Exchange Services. She is currently the Commissioning Development Worker for the Substance Misuse Advisory Service, a unit established within the UK Department of Health.

Wayne Blankenship was the Prevention Coordinator for Adult Gay/Bisexual Men at the San Francisco AIDS Foundation from 1991-1997. He also served as Education Coordinator for the Tucson AIDS Project, 1989-1991, where he developed the MEN ALOUD campaign, exported to over fifty American cities. Currently, Mr. Blankenship serves as the Program Director at the Zen Hospice Project in San Francisco.

Michael Bochow is a research fellow at Intersofia, Berlin (Institute for Applied Interdisciplinary Research in Social Problems). Since 1987 he has been commissioned by the Ministry of Health in Germany to conduct nationwide studies of HIV risk behavior among gay and bisexual men. In addition, he lends his expertise to research planning and development concerning HIV/AIDS prevention at the national level in France. His article was translated into English by Michael T. Wright.

Peter Davies is Professor of Sociology of Health and Director of Research in the School of Health Studies at the University of Portsmouth. He is a Director of Sigma Research and author of *Images of Social Stratification*, Sage 1985 and co-author with Ford Hickson, Peter Weatherburn and Andrew Hunt of *Sex, Gay Men & AIDS*, 1993. He is also joint editor with Peter Aggleton and Graham Hart of the *Social Aspects of AIDS* series published by Taylor & Francis.

Ford Hickson is a Senior Research Fellow with Sigma Research where he has been the principle researcher on a variety of projects, notably research into Male Rape. He is co-author with Peter Davies, Peter Weatherburn and Andrew Hunt of *Sex, Gay Men & AIDS*, Taylor & Francis, 1993. He is currently managing the Research and Development component of the

Community HIV/AIDS Prevention Strategy (CHAPS), the national gay men's HIV prevention strategy funded by the UK Department of Health.

Peter Keogh is Senior Research Fellow at Sigma Research at the University of Portsmouth in the United Kingdom, where he has been involved in numerous studies focusing on HIV transmission among gay and bisexual men. Research interests include community responses to HIV prevention; community representations of HIV positive gay men in relation to individual safer sex strategies; perceptions of partners' HIV status and non-verbally negotiated sexual encounters; and sexual networks of and sexual meanings for HIV positive gay men.

Rommel Mendès-Leite is a sociologist and social anthropologist affiliated with the Laboratoire d'Anthropologie Sociale of the École des Hautes Études en Sciences Sociales (LAS-EHESS) in Paris. He is also an associate researcher at the Institut National de Santé et de Recherche Médicale (INSERM), Unit 158. His primary interests are the discrepancies between the sexual practices of men who have sex with men and their socio-sexual behaviors; the construction of gay rationales; and HIV prevention. His latest book is *Bisexualité, le dernier tabou* (Paris, Calmann-Lévy, 1996). His paper is based on research made possible by support from the *Agece Nationale de Researches sur le Sida (ANRS)* in France and the *Conselho National de Desenvolvimento Cientifico e Tecnologico (CNPq)* in Brazil. The interviews in the paper were conducted in collaboration with Neila Mendès-Lopes as part of an ANRS project, *La Construction sociale des sexualités en Europe du Sud,* directed by Marie-Elizabeth Handman. The author is very grateful to Pierre-Oliver de Busscher, Michael Bochow, Yves Souterrand, Marie-Elizabeth Handman, Françoise Zonabend, Teresa Del Valle, Jean Jamin, Christian Deom and Catherine Deschamps.

David Nimmons has been active in community-based HIV prevention in New York since 1982. He was past president of the New York City Lesbian & Gay Community Center and former Managing Director of Education and Chief of Staff at New York's Gay Men's Health Crisis. Currently he is working with the Center for AIDS Prevention Studies to investigate the role of altruistic and communal motivators in gay men's sexual safety decisions. Mr. Nimmons is a Revson Fellow at Columbia University.

Eric Rofes is the author of the book *Reviving the Tribe: Regenerating Gay Men's Sexuality and Culture in the Ongoing Epidemic* (The Haworth Press, Inc.) and of the forthcoming *Dry Bones Breath: Gay Men Creating Post-AIDS Identities and Cultures* (The Haworth Press, Inc.). He has served as the executive director of the Los Angeles Gay and Lesbian Community Services Center and San Francisco's Shanti Project. He is currently an instructor at the University of California at Berkeley's Graduate School of Education, where he is a doctoral student in Social and Cultural Studies. His essay was adapted from a speech given at a conference hosted by the National Minority AIDS Council and the Centers for Disease Control and Prevention, (C.D.C.), Atlanta, GA.

B. R. Simon Rosser is an associate professor and licensed psychologist at the Program in Human Sexuality, Department of Family Practice and Community Health, Medical School, University of Minnesota. Originally from New Zealand, Dr. Rosser has conducted HIV prevention research in four countries, and has published two books and over 60 research articles on aspects of HIV prevention and human sexuality. Currently, he is principal investigator of a Centers for Disease Control and Prevention (C.D.C.) funded study examining new approaches to HIV prevention targeting men who have sex with men, and serves on the Minnesota Health Commissioner's Task Force on HIV and STD Prevention. An earlier version of his article was published in the newsletter of the National Lesbian and Gay Health Association. The author would like to acknowledge the involvement of the participants from the caucus, and also Jerry Calumn, Hart Roussel, Michael Wright, Dr. Joyce Hunter, and the Board of the NLGHA in the development of this report.

Theo G. M. Sandfort is a social psychologist who works as a researcher at the Center for Gay and Lesbian Studies at Utrecht University and is research coordinator at the Netherlands Institute for Social Sexological Research (NISSO, Utrecht). The research he directs focuses on determinants of HIV-preventive behavior in gay men as well as in the general population. He is also involved in studies monitoring behavioral changes and assessing the impact of small and large scale interventions aimed at promoting safer sex behavior. In addition to HIV/AIDS-related issues, he studies aspects of gay and lesbian lives, including coming out processes, life styles, relationships and discrimination.

Marie-Ange Schiltz is a researcher at the CNRS (Centre National de la Recherche Scientifique) in Paris, and a doctoral candidate at the University of Paris. Since 1985 she has worked on the annual national study of lifestyles and adaptation to AIDS among gay and bisexual men in France. She has published in *Actes de la Recherche en Sciences Sociales, Anthropologie et Société*, and *AIDS Care*. Her article was translated into English by Marguerite Le Clézio.

Marty P. N. van Kerkhof is a sociologist, freelance researcher and journalist. He is working in the fields of AIDS (prevention and care) and sexuality. Recently he published a book on bisexuality.

Peter Weatherburn is Research Manager with Sigma Research where he has been the principle researcher on a variety of projects, notably research into behaviourally bisexual men. He is co-author with Peter Davies, Ford Hickson and Andrew Hunt of *Sex, Gay Men & AIDS*, Taylor & Francis, 1993. He is currently researching the impact of new HIV treatments on people with AIDS.

Michael T. Wright served as a consultant and as Director of International Relations at the Deutsche AIDS-Hilfe, the national German AIDS organization, from 1994-1997. He has been involved in HIV prevention work since 1984, having served as a psychotherapist, program manager, clinical supervisor, researcher, workshop leader and consultant. He is a graduate of the Harvard School of Public Health and is currently conducting research at the Institute for Prevention and Psychosocial Research at The Free University in Berlin, Germany. He wishes to acknowledge the invaluable assistance of Norbet Broemme in organizing the Chorin symposium. He can be contacted via e-mail at: mtwright@compuserve.com

Onno de Zwart is HIV/AIDS Policy Coordinator at the Rotterdam Municipal Health Service, where he has also served as assistant coordinator of the Multi-City Action Plan on AIDS, a network of fifteen European cities. As a researcher in the Department of Gay and Lesbian Studies at Utrecht University, he focused on Dutch HIV prevention policy directed at men who have sex with men. Together with Marty P. N. Van Kerkhof, Mr. de Zwart conducted an in-depth study on the meaning of anal sex for gay men. The research described in this paper was carried out at the Department of Gay and Lesbian Studies, Utrecht University. The study was financially supported by the Netherlands Foundation for Preventive Medicine (grant 92011). The authors wish to thank André Steffens and Michael T. Wright for their useful comments.

Index

Aarburg, Hans-Peter von, 128
ACON (AIDS Council of New South Wales), 49
Acquired immunodeficiency syndrome. *See* AIDS
Activism, 157
Age, HIV infection rate and, 51-52
Aggleton, Peter, 8-9
AIDS
    lessons learned, 134-135
    unlearned lessons, 135-137
    word choice and, 15
AIDS Council of New South Wales (ACON), 49
AIDS Service Organizations (ASOs), 147
Altruism. *See* Prevention altruism
Anal intercourse, 90
    condom use and, in Germany, 44-46
    factors influencing having, 93-100
    role decisions for, 95
    scenarios, 96-100
    trust as prerequisite for, 93-94
    types of partnership and, in Germany, 42-44
Anti-retrovirals, 47
ASOs. *See* AIDS Service Organizations (ASOs)

Blankenship, Wayne, 2
Bochow, Michael, 2
Bonding, unprotected sex and, 77

Chorin document, 2-6
    goals, 2
    participants, 2-3
    topics, 3-6
Coates, Tom, 3
Condoms
    fellatio and, 26,112-113
    in intimate scenarios, 97-98
    messages for use, 55
    in physical scenarios, 96-97
    in power scenarios, 99-100
    in reciprocal scenarios, 98-99
    use of, in France, 26-27
    use of, in Germany, 44-46
Context, importance of, 135
Contextualization, 40,55-56
Coping strategies, 27-28
Coupling, 12
Cruising, and HIV risk, 29
Culture
    as determinant for sexual behavior, 12-14
    sexual interaction and, 11

Dangerous sex, psychology of, 7-8
Deception, 14
Decision-making, sexual, 14
Desire
    cultural definitions of, 124-125
    in HIV prevention research, 13
Deutsche AIDS-Hilfe, 2
Drug companies, ethical obligations of, 148

Enquête Presse Gaie (France), 20. *See also* Gay Press Survey (France)

Faithfulness, 108-109
Fantasy, 49
Fast-track licensing, impact on information dissemination, 148
Fellatio, condom use and, 26, 112-113
Fixed personality traits, 11
Forgotten populations, 145
France
   AIDS cases in, 21-22
   changes in gay sexual behavior, 20
   HIV prevention landmarks, 21

Gay Press Survey (France), 20
   adjustment to HIV risk, 25-26
   conclusions, 30-32
   condom use, 26-27
   continuing risk behavior, 28-29
   coping strategies, 27-28
   cruising associated with HIV risk, 29-30
   methodology, 22-23
   perceptions of social acceptance and diversity of lifestyle, 23-25
Gay Press Survey (Germany)
   condom use, 44-46
   methodology, 40-41
   risk-minimizing strategies results, 49-51
   types of partnership results, 42-49
Grounded theory approach, 91-92

Health Belief Model, 8
Health promotion materials, 67-71
HIV
   drug resistant strains of, 145
   gay men diagnosed with, 61-65
   imaginary protection mechanisms, 106-107
   infection rate of, and age, in Germany, 51-52
   levels of discourse on, 70-71
   as long-term manageable illness, 144
   men who know or assume themselves to be uninfected with, 65-67
   new testing methodologies, 145
   risk-minimizing strategies, 50-51
HIV/AIDS
   impact of research on HIV prevention workers, 151-158
   lessons learned, 134-135
   unlearned lessons, 135-137
   word choice and, 15
HIV medication development, indirect effects of, 147
HIV prevention, 5
   changes in, 157
   Chorin document for, 2-6
   and cultural contexts, 106
   effect of hope in a cure on, 144-145
   factors affecting implementing programs for, 6
   funding challenges for, 145-146
   future directions, 137-138
   HIV as manageable illness and, 144
   impact of research, 147-148
   impact of viral load and new medications on, 145
   landmarks in France, 21
   manipulation of techniques for, 104
   models, 55
   programs, 76,77
   promotion materials for, 67-71
   structural problem of, 54-55
   zero risk objectives, 29
HIV prevention workers, impact of HIV/AIDS research on, 151-158

HIV-testing, risk minimizing
    strategies and, 50-51
Homosexuality, study of, 20
Hope, in a cure, 144-145
Human immunodeficiency virus. *See*
    HIV

Identity, meaning of sexual acts and, 5
Imaginary protections, 14,104-107
    benefits of theory, 117-118
    and Others, 116-117
Incidents, planned and unplanned,
    65-66
Individuals as research unit, sex
    research and, 11
Information dissemination, 148
Intimacy, 12
Intimate scenarios, for anal sex, 97-98

Kippax, Susan, 40

Limited rationality, 110
Loneliness, unprotected sex and, 77
Love, 13,48-49
Low viral load, 157-158

Meaning, symbolic, 14
Medications, new, 145,146
Mendès-Leite, Rommel, 3
Multiculturalism, 15

Negotiated safety, 53-54,66,77
Negotiation, sexual, 63-64
Nimmons, Dave, 3

Odets, Walt, 127
Others, imaginary protections and,
    116-117

Partnerships, sexual
    number of, and risk behavior, in
        Germany, 46-49
    types of, and anal intercourse, in
        Germany, 42-43
    types of, and risk behavior, in
        Germany, 42-43
Permanent relationships, 49
Person as static entity, sex research
    and, 11
Pharmaceutical companies, ethical
    obligations of, 148
Physical scenarios, for anal sex,
    96-97
Pientka, Ludger, 39
Planned incidents, 65-66
Pleasure, 13
Pollak, Michael, 20
Populations, forgotten, 145
Post-HIV exposure prophylaxis, 147
Power
    role of, in sexual encounters, 13
    scenarios, for anal sex, 99-100
Prevention. *See* HIV prevention
Prevention altruism
    evidence for, 78-82
    testing and applying, 82-83
Prevention concepts, 106
Prophylaxis, post-HIV exposure, 147
Protease inhibitors, 145
Protected sex. *See also* Safer sex;
        Unprotected sex scenarios
    of anal sex and, 96-100

Rational decision making, sex as, 10
Rationality, limited, 110
Rational models, of sexual behavior,
    103-104
Reciprocal scenarios, for anal sex,
    98-99
Re-infection, 79
Relapse, 8,29-30
Relationships, 49
Residual risk, 20

Risk, as positive concept, 128
Risk behavior, 20
   frequency of, 30
   number of partners and, in Germany, 46-49
   patterns, 147
   types of partnership and, in Germany, 43-44
   of younger German gay men, 51-53
Risk factor love, 13, 48-49
Risk factor model, fallacies of, 39
Risk factors, 8
Risk management, 103-104
   goal of, 32
   structural problem of, 54-55
Risk minimization concept, 40
Risk-minimizing strategies
   HIV-testing and, 50-51
   patterns of, 49-50
Rofes, Eric, 3
Role decisions, for anal sex, 95
Romantic dimensions, of sexuality, 13
Rosenbrock, Rolf, 3, 8

Safer sex, 8, 67
   goal of, 76
   strategy, 50
   symbolic meanings of, 125-126
Safer sex research, 7-8
   European trends, 7-16
   expanding paradigm for, 9-10
   themes, 10-11
Schiltz, Marie-Ange, 3
Scripts, sexual, 91
Selective strategies, 49-50
Self-deception, 14
Self-interest paradigm of HIV prevention, 76-78
Sex
   cultural definitions of, 124-125
   psychology of dangerous, 7-8
   social context of, 11

Sex research
   expanded paradigm implications, 14-16
   expanding the horizons of future, 11-14
   person as static entity for, 11
Sexual acts
   factors influencing people to engage in, 4-5
   meaning of, and identity, 5
Sexual behavior, 8, 11
   changes in, by gays in France, 20
   rationality models and, 103-104
Sexual decision-making, 14
Sexuality, word choice for, 15
Sexual negotiation, 63-64
Sexual partnerships. *See* Partnerships, sexual
Sexual scripts, 91
Social imagery of sexualities, 106
Social Learning theory, 8
Steady relationship strategy, 50
Symbolic meaning, 14

Time, sex research and, 11
Transgendered persons, 145
Trust, as prerequisite for anal sex, 93-94

Undetectable virus, 157-158
Unplanned incidents, 65
Unprotected anal sex, 90
Unprotected sex, 8
   bonding and, 77
   loneliness and, 77
   and viral mutation, 145
Unsafe sex. *See* Unprotected sex

Viral apartheid, 129
Viral load
   impact of, on HIV prevention, 145
   low, and transmissibility, 157-158

Viral mutation, unprotected sex and, 145

Weikert, Matthias, 3
Word choice, for sexuality, 15
Wright, Michael, 3

Zero risk objective, 29
Zwart, Onno de, 3

Haworth DOCUMENT DELIVERY SERVICE

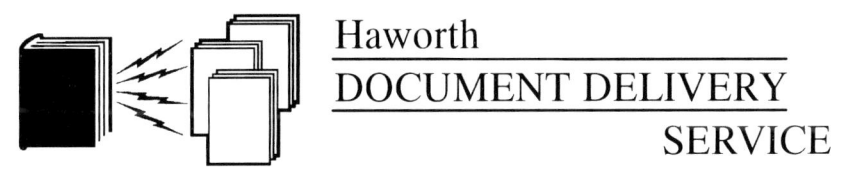

This valuable service provides a single-article order form for any article from a Haworth journal.

- *Time Saving:* No running around from library to library to find a specific article.
- *Cost Effective:* All costs are kept down to a minimum.
- *Fast Delivery:* Choose from several options, including same-day FAX.
- *No Copyright Hassles:* You will be supplied by the original publisher.
- *Easy Payment:* Choose from several easy payment methods.

Open Accounts Welcome for . . .
- Library Interlibrary Loan Departments
- Library Network/Consortia Wishing to Provide Single-Article Services
- Indexing/Abstracting Services with Single Article Provision Services
- Document Provision Brokers and Freelance Information Service Providers

MAIL or *FAX* THIS ENTIRE ORDER FORM TO:

Haworth Document Delivery Service
The Haworth Press, Inc.
10 Alice Street
Binghamton, NY 13904-1580

or FAX: 1-800-895-0582
or CALL: 1-800-429-6784
9am-5pm EST

PLEASE SEND ME PHOTOCOPIES OF THE FOLLOWING SINGLE ARTICLES:

1) Journal Title: _____
    Vol/Issue/Year: _____ Starting & Ending Pages: _____
    Article Title: _____

2) Journal Title: _____
    Vol/Issue/Year: _____ Starting & Ending Pages: _____
    Article Title: _____

3) Journal Title: _____
    Vol/Issue/Year: _____ Starting & Ending Pages: _____
    Article Title: _____

4) Journal Title: _____
    Vol/Issue/Year: _____ Starting & Ending Pages: _____
    Article Title: _____

(See other side for Costs and Payment Information)

COSTS: Please figure your cost to order quality copies of an article.

1. Set-up charge per article: $8.00
    ($8.00 × number of separate articles) _____

2. Photocopying charge for each article:
    1-10 pages: $1.00 _____

    11-19 pages: $3.00 _____

    20-29 pages: $5.00 _____

    30+ pages: $2.00/10 pages _____

3. Flexicover (optional): $2.00/article _____

4. Postage & Handling: US: $1.00 for the first article/
    $.50 each additional article _____

    Federal Express: $25.00 _____

    Outside US: $2.00 for first article/
    $.50 each additional article _____

5. Same-day FAX service: $.50 per page _____

GRAND TOTAL: _____

METHOD OF PAYMENT: (please check one)

❏ Check enclosed   ❏ Please ship and bill. PO # _____
    (sorry we can ship and bill to bookstores only! All others must pre-pay)

❏ Charge to my credit card: ❏ Visa; ❏ MasterCard; ❏ Discover;
    ❏ American Express;

Account Number: _____ Expiration date: _____

Signature: X _____

Name: _____ Institution: _____

Address: _____

_____

City: _____ State: _____ Zip: _____

Phone Number: _____ FAX Number: _____

MAIL or *FAX* THIS ENTIRE ORDER FORM TO:

Haworth Document Delivery Service	**or FAX:** 1-800-895-0582
The Haworth Press, Inc.	**or CALL:** 1-800-429-6784
10 Alice Street	(9am-5pm EST)
Binghamton, NY 13904-1580	